VICTIM NO MORE

How Forgiving Dad Turned Victim to Victor

Charles J. Huff

EABooks Publishing
Your Partner In Publishing

ISBN: 978-1-955309-33-2
LCCN: 2023902763
Cover photo: iStock/NiseriN
Author photo from the author's personal collection
Design: Robin Black

Published by EA Books Publishing, a division of
Living Parables of Central Florida, Inc. a 501c3

EABooksPublishing.com

DEDICATION

I want to honor those who have had such an impact on my life to bring a message and hope.

First, I dedicate this story to my family—past and present—who have helped shape me into who I am today.

The greatest thanks goes to my wife Cindy who stood by me, giving me comfort and encouragement along the way, especially when she didn't know how deeply I had to dig in my past to create a new future.

Finally, a special tribute goes to Ginger Kolbaba who, as my coach and editor, kept me working on polishing my draft. Every time I felt like giving up, she sent me the right words of encouragement when I needed them most.

CONTENTS

THE BURGUNDY PHOTO ALBUM

I ran my fingers across the raised image on the burgundy photo album cover. A black shoestring on the left side tied together the covers and the inch or more of black construction paper trapped inside to create a book. The front cover no longer lay flat. Instead, it arched over pages swollen with the treasure trove of memories.

At seven years old, after years of being laid up with my legs in casts—a result of procedures to correct severe club feet—looking through the old family snapshots became one of my favorite ways to occupy myself and pass the time. Besides changing the shape of my feet, the casts also conditioned me to sit still, which meant the albums became my go-to place. I paused on each page, remembering what Mom had told me about each picture.

I stared at one photo and wondered about the family looking back at me. What were their lives like back then? Mom said the trio was her, Dad, and my brother when he was about two years old. I looked at each face and saw only hints of them. The man stood lanky with hair parted on one side. His face seemed long and angular. The dad I knew had a square face and a round stomach. His hair was short, cut in a flattop. The woman resembled Mom, but so much had changed in the nearly fifteen years since they'd had the picture taken. I leaned over to inspect the differences. The man holding the boy looked proud of his little man. The couple stood close to each other. They looked happy.

I touched the image of the boy. *Why couldn't that have been me? Why did I have only the evil dad to remember?*

As I lingered over the picture, I recalled a time when we arrived home after I had my casts replaced with a new set. I must have been four years old when Dad pulled into the driveway and stopped near the front door of our house. I cringed when he lifted me from the back-seat of the car. I hoped he wasn't mad at me because I couldn't walk. I didn't want him to be. *I'm sorry, Dad.*

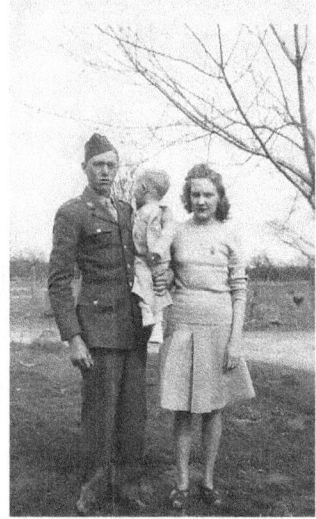

I longed for any show of affection or caring.

For a brief moment, a sense of delight slipped in and wrapped me as a shield against my fears. I was in Daddy's arms, just like my brother was in this picture. My lungs filled with the scent of his Old Spice cologne. His arms supported me under and behind, against his side, and my arms were about his neck. *Why hadn't someone taken a picture of us then?*

We stepped into the house, and he set me on the floor. The moment was over. Gone forever. It was the last time I felt Dad's arms around me, gentle and protective, even if it was only out of duty.

I shook myself out of the daydream and continued looking through the album. There was Dad in the army—in training, in New Guinea, in the Philippines, in Japan. My brother, Kenny, and Mom back on Grandma and Grandpa Mulvaney's farm.

I flipped the page and studied the smiling face of Dad home from the war, visiting army buddies.

Then I was born.

The rest of the pages were empty.

CHAPTER 1

INTO THIS I CAME

Like wisps of smoke, my earliest memories are short and fleeting. They leave me wondering how it's possible things so small have the strength to forge me into who I am. I can't help but question what other things happened that I don't remember. They might be as important as the clear snippets my mind's eye has captured. I imagine them floating around in my subconscious, waiting until conditions are right to let me glimpse their flittering shadows. Do I want to see the secrets they hold? Will they reveal more hurts? Or will I find the loving family I hoped for?

The picture in the photo album whispered to me that our family was happy once. It wasn't today. I caught my tears before they touched the pages. Dad had come home drunk again. This time he had whipped me for plugging the toilet by using too much toilet paper.

As I knelt beside the coffee table before the open album, too sore to sit down, I wondered why my dad was not more like Jim Anderson in the popular television show *Father Knows Best*. He could be stern and loving at the same time. Most important, he never struck anyone. The fathers in *Make Room for Daddy, Ozzie and Harriet, Leave It to Beaver*, and *Lassie* also portrayed the type of dad I wanted. The type of family I wanted.

But we were broken. In my earliest memories, I knew something was wrong in our family. We didn't match the ideals portrayed almost nightly on television shows. I also believed we didn't match at least half our extended family. Although three uncles drank beer heavily like Dad, the other seven didn't drink at all, as far as I had seen. At the family gatherings, I watched how they treated one another and especially how they treated their kids. How their kids treated them also did not escape my notice. They seemed kind to one another and happy. I say seemed because in the gatherings, Dad made our family seem in good form, too.

What happened to our family? I wondered. I mean, if Dad was always like this—drunk and mean—why did Mom marry him? If he wasn't, what changed him? And could we get the first version of him back?

I actually knew very little of Dad. He went to work. After work he went to a bar. He came home and often whipped me. Then he went to bed. I never knew what he could do with his mind and his hands when he had purpose.

Mom, on the other hand, was always busy. She sewed her own clothes; painted the walls when redecorating; grew a large garden; cooked; and canned or froze fruits, preserves, and vegetables. She even did some carpentry.

Had Dad ever been that industrious? Was their life together always like what I saw every day? If not, what caused it to unravel, and when? I felt a lump form in my throat, and I tried to swallow it down. *Was I the cause?*

Over the years, I asked Mom to tell me stories of what life used to be like for her and Dad, sometimes asking for the same ones so I could remember more details.

"Well, this house we live in used to be only two rooms," she recalled. "One house we lived in before the war was on Yard's Road. Your dad worked on the railroad at the time, so it was close to work for him."

She called it their cardboard house. The housing demand during the oil boom in the nineteen thirties and forties called for quick, inexpensive construction. The cardboard house had thin walls constructed of pressed-paper fiberboard panels less than a quarter of an inch thick nailed to two-by-two studs.

Mom scowled as she described the construction. She knew what proper building materials and methods were. Those homes violated every one of the standards. Mom surprised me when she paused in thought, then sat back and chuckled. "I was upset that your dad had not come home on time."

I reasoned by that comment Dad began being absent very early but had not started out that way. I leaned forward to refocus on Mom's story.

"I had plenty of time to figure out a scheme to get him to realize what I went through every time he did that. When I heard the sound of tires crunching gravel outside, I hid in one of the cardboard closets. My plan was to make him miss me to the point of getting worried, then I would hop out and surprise him.

"I heard the door open and your dad call out, 'Norma.' I covered my mouth. I wouldn't let my snickers give away my hiding place. Again he called out, 'Norma, where are you?' His tone told me my plan was working out fine. I held my breath as your dad's footsteps passed close. He looked in all the rooms, but not in the closet. I was wondering how long I should make him wait, when I heard him start talking to somebody."

I sat back. "What?" The twist in the story made me laugh. "Who was there? What did he say?"

Mom crossed her arms and held them close to her chest. "I don't know who it was. All I heard him say was, 'Maybe she went to see her sister. She should be back soon. Want a beer while you wait?'"

The beer part sounded familiar to me, so I nodded.

"Joe had brought someone home with him, and I had trapped myself. There was no way I wanted to pop out of the closet then. I had no idea who was with him, and I didn't want to have to explain. I hoped he didn't hear me gasp. My legs grew tired as I waited for them to leave. Tiredness gave way to hurting, then numbness settled in as I tried to stay perfectly still. I had no idea how long I was in the closet, but my stomach told me it was well after supper time."

I shook my head. "Wow. I can't believe you were able to stay in there that long and that no one heard you."

"Well, finally, your dad said, 'I don't know what happened to Norma. I guess we'll have to try this another night. Sorry. You would have liked her cooking.'"

"He brought the person home for supper?" I asked and she nodded. "Then what happened?"

"Chairs scooted. Footsteps. The front door opened and closed. I stayed in my hiding spot, listening for sounds that would tell me they both were not coming back in. Muffled voices. Two car doors slammed. Then the car engine revved and tires crunched gravel again. He was giving his friend a ride somewhere and would be back later. Only then did I open the closet door and uncurl myself into the room."

I leaned farther forward. "What did Dad say when he found out?"

"He laughed at me. Said it served me right."

I smiled at the glimpse of the family life I wanted, the happy family in the photograph. Mom and Dad used to have fun and enjoy each other's antics. Oh, how I wanted them to be that way again—every day, not in rare moments.

The more questions I asked, the more Mom revealed. She filled in big gaps of time as she told me of life before I came along. Ten years before me, the family started with Mom, Dad, and an older sister named Carolyn, who was born in February 1940. She died of scarlet fever six months later. Mom caught it from her and nearly died, but her fever broke on the day of Carolyn's funeral. Some family members held up the tiny casket to the bedroom window for Mom to see. She screamed at them, "Why didn't you let me die too?"

As Mom said those words, her eyes clouded over, and she seemed lost in her thoughts. Her mood changed to sadness.

Though I never knew my sister, the loss still overshadowed our family. Each Memorial Day, Mom and I placed flowers in front of her cast-iron marker in the cemetery. I watched as Mom's eyes took on a sad, faraway stare, as if observing her most painful six months.

I'd discovered a couple mementos of Carolyn in Mom and Dad's cedar chest—a newborn photo, a funeral photo. Sometimes I would look at those photos and remember Mom's story. Those were all that remained of her. Whenever an infant died in the area, I saw that same look cross Mom's face. She was sure those who lost a child right after birth could not know the depths of loss after having held and fed the infant for months before it died.

In February 1942, Mom gave birth to my brother, Kenny. "As he got older, he asked your dad and me for a baby brother to play with." Her eyes grew tender as she nodded at me. "He didn't seem as excited as I expected he would be when we told him we were going to have another baby. I guess too many years had passed."

I bit the inside of my cheek. That must have been why he never seemed to want me around or invite me to play with him. He always acted like life would be better if he had been an only child. *Why does there have to be eight years between us? Then maybe we could be a happy family.*

"And then—" Mom's sweet voice cut into my thoughts.

"Then I was born!" I said, delightedly, turning my mind off my brother and onto the more interesting part of the story. March 1950, I became the last member of our little family and the only one in my immediate family to be born in a hospital.

Mom never had time to answer all of my questions, so I would get parts of stories and then have to wait until later. As I got older, I learned to take advantage of certain summer activities to ask Mom for more stories. Although I hated working in the garden, I didn't mind helping prep fruit and vegetables for canning or for the evening meal. Snapping green beans always suited me for getting Mom to talk.

"What happened when I was born?" I asked one day.

"I sent Kenny to stay with my mom and dad on the farm just before you were born. I had no one with me at the hospital."

"Where was Dad?"

"At the bar getting drunk."

Mom's answer struck me as though she expected nothing else of Dad, but it wasn't without a hint of disgust and anger.

I had more than a little anger triggered. Why would any father-to-be abandon his wife in such a time? Was he drinking in celebration or drowning his thoughts of not wanting me? Whatever his reason, he left Mom to face alone the news that I was born with two severely clubbed feet.

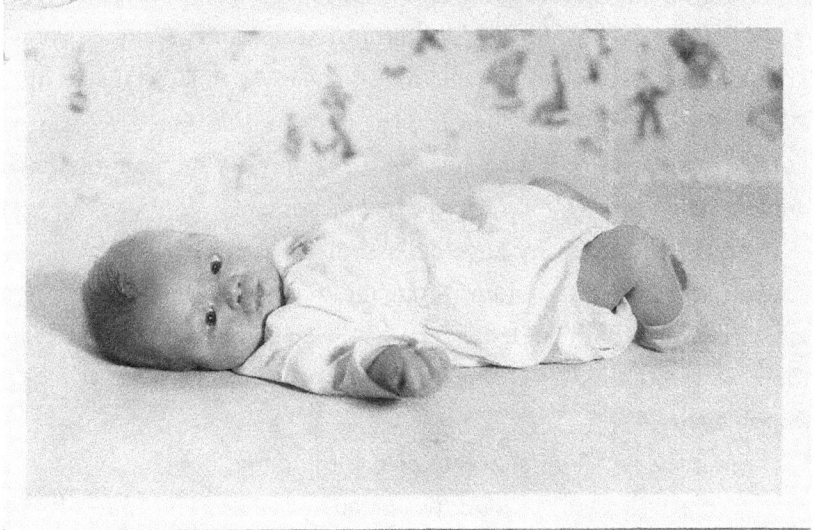

Feet were curled (clubbed) too much to show in picture.

I didn't ask if Dad ever made himself available to help make the immediate decisions on what was going to be done for my condition. I never thought of it because I was still too angry at what he had done, too hurt that he didn't care to be there when I was born, and too filled with wonder at Mom's strength in it all.

"So what was I like as a baby?"

"Actually, I saw very little of you for your first three years. We didn't have insurance or the money to afford what you needed. The doctor recommended Shriner's Hospital in St. Louis. They specialized in birth defects and took on cases like ours free of charge. They had one requirement. We drop you off there and not visit until they would call us to pick you up."

A slight tremble in her voice as she shared this made me wonder what troubled her still. Did leaving me without being able to visit upset her? Or did I remind her of six-month-old Carolyn being taken from her without so much as a touch or a goodbye?

I looked down at my feet. The black orthopedic shoes were expensive. I knew that by overhearing Mom and Dad talking about how to pay for them. Too bad they didn't have some style added to them. They did little to

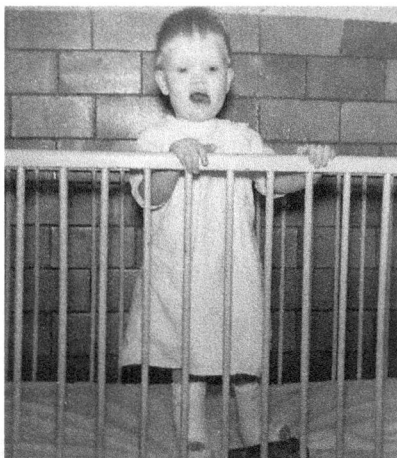

A mother of another child in my hospital ward took this picture and sent it to my mom with a note of compassion since I never received visitors.

hide the high arch that caused my feet to be short for my height.

"What did the doctors do?" I couldn't remember, naturally, what my feet were like from birth. Mom tried to describe them, but I couldn't picture it.

She explained that for those first three years, doctors bent the bones and locked them into position with casts to reshape my feet and straighten my legs. Without the casts, my feet would curve back toward their twisted form. Because I was so young and was growing so fast, they changed the casts frequently in the beginning. That's why they kept me in the hospital instead of checking me in and out every little bit.

Mom set her pan of green beans on the table. "I'll be right back."

I craned my neck to watch as she headed toward her bedroom. I heard what sounded like the lid to her cedar chest open and close. She returned to the kitchen and handed me a plastic key with its plastic ring. "This was your teething ring."

The muscles in my back tightened with the thought of biting hard plastic with swollen gums. After a bit, I handed it back to her. "Why didn't the doctors just do surgery?"

"They couldn't before your bones were nearly done growing, so their goal was to lessen the amount of correction needed. I guess you were about two when we learned that a hospital in Chicago offered the same no- or minimal-cost services, and it allowed visitors."

Unfortunately, being more than twice the distance away, however, kept my parents away just the same. Mom said Dad's brother Keith promised either he or his wife would check on me while I was there.

I had more questions to ask, but Mom glanced up at the clock on the wall. "We better get started canning these beans or I will still be doing them while trying to get supper at the same time."

When she said *we*, she meant herself. I couldn't be much help, so she shooed me out of the kitchen.

Once outside, I walked around to the shady side of the house to escape the hot sun. Sitting against the house foundation, I began to pick and eat some sheep sorrel that grew wild in our yard. I loved that sour herb, probably more than green apples. I continued thinking about what Mom had told me, trying desperately to remember as far back as I could.

After nearly three years in hospitals with few visits home, the day came when I received casts that could stay on longer than a month, which meant I could go home for a while. That's where my memory picked up.

At the end of my time at home, my heels stuck out of the casts. Since I couldn't walk, I had to scoot everywhere. And my continual scooting wore off that heel part.

I also graduated out of the toddler treatments of constant casts. Instead, I had periods during which I wore prescription shoes or wore shoes on the wrong feet to help force the arch and toes outward.

That summer, during one of the times I was without casts, Mom and Dad added two bedrooms, a joined closet, and a bathroom to our house, more than doubling its size. Mom told me I was three when they built the addition. Because I couldn't remember being in the hospitals, Mom's dateline surprised me. But that also explained why my recall of that time were only sketchy snippets. The biggest change for me—besides having my own bed—was no more going to the outhouse. While they were still common in rural America, I was glad to see ours go into history. It would be another ten years or more before my dad's aunts stopped using theirs.

The bedrooms and bath additions helped Mom a lot, I'm sure. It made taking me to the bathroom much easier—for her and me. Being afraid of the dark made night trips to the outhouse out of the question for me, and I hated the chamber pot.

Without the casts, I had to wear a brace to bed. That was the worst treatment I had to endure. The brace was a flat bar with shoes attached at each end for my feet. It held my legs and feet into the position necessary for everything to properly align and grow while I slept.

"Stop kicking. You know the doctor said you have to wear this."

"I don't see it makes any difference." I tried moving away from Mom—even sliding off the opposite side of the bed.

"You won't see immediate results. This is a slow process. Do you want to wear shoes like the one the man in town wears? He has a clubfoot, too."

I gave up. I knew I was never going to win this fight.

Mom talked softly as she slipped both feet into shoes on the bar and tied the shoestrings. She talked of what we would be doing the next day and how much better my feet would be in time.

"I hate this because I like to sleep on my side."

"Here, let me help you turn over and see if you can twist into a comfortable position." She held the covers high and helped me roll my legs and hip over. On my stomach, I was able to roll my shoulders enough to be somewhat on my side.

"That's better. Thanks, Mom."

"Now try to go to sleep. Good night."

I knew how much my mother did for our family. And I knew I had become one more burden for her. Especially if I needed to go to the bathroom in the night. Thankfully that was rare, at least I think it was.

For a while, the benefits of our new indoor plumbing outweighed what we had before. But it didn't take long to discover its drawbacks. In the outhouse, a person could use any amount of toilet paper they wanted. Too much in the toilet caused a problem. When I flushed it, the water kept rising until it splashed onto the floor. Mom heard and rushed in to start plunging it until it went down. Then she cleaned up the mess.

I tried to keep the amount used low, but I wasn't always successful. One unsuccessful attempt happened one night after Dad came home drunk. He heard the commotion and got up to see what had happened. He started yelling about causing problems in the sewer—maybe costly repairs and other things that I knew nothing about, but that were important to him. He snapped out his belt and started beating on me, telling me I better not do that again.

"Stop," Mom kept telling him. "Let's just get this cleaned up."

But that scene happened enough times to make me hesitant to use the bathroom at all. From the time I was five to seven years old, I became plagued with constipation. I hoped an uncontrollable urge would strike during the day when I could run for the outhouse. But soon, the bathroom became a greater terror than the dark.

I couldn't control my urges and no amount of time sitting on the toilet ever accomplished a thing for me. A missed opportunity could go for hours before the urge hit me again. By then, my movement would not go down the toilet. Dad had to plunge the toilet while Mom cleaned up the overflow.

When they had finished, Dad took off his belt and whipped me. Time after time. Whether too much toilet paper or a bout of constipation, the toilet would not flush completely and start backing up. And I got a thrashing. Sometimes, I had to sleep on my stomach because my backside hurt too much to lie on it. Purple welts striped my back, buttocks, and thighs. If I turned just right, I could see some of them in the mirror. It took little imagination to know what the rest of me looked like.

I tried to keep from going to the bathroom out of fear it would trigger another beating. That did little more than increase my constipation.

"The next time this happens, I will make you pull your stuff out of the toilet with your hands and throw it outside!" Dad said, winding his belt back through his pants loops and rebuckling it.

I determined not to let it happen again, but of course, that was impossible. And the next time it happened, I panicked.

Dad stood over me with his hands on his hips. "You know what I said would happen if you did this again. Now pull it out."

As I started to cry, Dad shifted his hands to his belt. Of all things Dad would remember he said when he was drunk, why did it have to be this one? I willed my tears to stop while I sat looking in the toilet and whimpered.

Mom tried to squeeze through the doorway, but Dad pushed her back out. He wasn't going to allow her to get me off the hook. After a few moments, she returned with an empty cardboard milk carton. "Here," she said, reaching around Dad. "Drop it in here."

Dad allowed that. I think he felt a sense of victory, but I perhaps more so. I avoided a whipping. I also learned that with a long, thin, but rigid tool, I could chop my waste into flushable pieces. Not the healthiest outcome, I know, but I survived.

That same summer, Dad butchered his last hog. While that freed up some of his time required by the farm, he never filled it with family time. He used his new freedom to spend the extra minutes and hours at a bar in town.

We had only one car, and Dad usually drove himself to work. Mom always said it was Dad's way of making sure she stayed at home. On the days Mom needed the family car to shop for groceries, do laundry, or run errands, she, Kenny, and I drove into town to pick Dad up from work.

Whether Dad got in the passenger side or made Mom scoot over so he could drive, the result was the same. "I want to stop at the tavern for a quick drink." Sometimes he said he needed to talk to someone about a matter. Most often he offered no excuse.

While Dad went inside, we waited in the car. The alley behind the tavern where Dad usually parked offered little for entertainment or imagination. Brick walls with louvered windows for fan ventilation and one door for each establishment. The lights on the back of the building shone bright enough at night to give some shadows.

"Mom, what kind of trees are those next to the building?"

"They are more like weeds that grow like trees. They are worthless. People call them Devil's Walking Sticks."

"What's in all those boxes, Mom?"

"Empty beer bottles."

"Really? What do they do with them?"

"They give them back to the bottling company for money. That's why you see your dad hauling his empty bottles back to the tavern. He gets paid for the bottles—or they cover the bottle recycling fee for the bottles he brings home."

"How much?"

"Each case is worth a little over a dollar."

"Look at how many boxes there are. That's a lot of money sitting there."

After an hour or more, Mom would decide to go into the tavern to see if she could coax Dad into leaving. She still had to fix supper for us once we got home, and it was getting late.

Kenny would be lost in his own world and his *Field and Stream* magazine, letting Mom and me chatter. With her gone, I turned my energy to him.

"Why don't you just look at the comic books you brought and be quiet?" he said, keeping his nose in his magazine.

"It's been too long. I'm tired. I want to go home."

"So do I, but there's nothing we can do but wait for when Dad decides to come out. It's still light enough for you to see your books, so look at them."

"I don't want to."

"Then why did you bring them?"

"I'm just tired of waiting."

"You have no idea what waiting on Dad is like. I've had to wait in the car all by myself in the winter. The car got colder and colder, but no Mom or Dad came out. One time they had to warm the car and scrape the windows before we could start home."

My eyes grew wide. "What did you do?"

"I read what I brought with me while there was enough light. I created games to distract me. They helped the time go by faster but could do nothing for the cold. Now look at your books and be quiet."

"Let me read you my favorite story." Unable to read yet, I launched into a story based in part on what I remembered others had read to me and mainly on what the pictures suggested to me.

"That's not what that says." Kenny stopped me when I had strayed so far from the written story that there was no hope of returning to it.

"Does too."

He sighed, sounding frustrated, then picked up one of my other comic books and turned his back to me. He was not going to be any more help for me that night.

Please, Mom and Dad, come out so we can go home.

More time passed before the back door of the tavern opened. Dad walked out in the lead, unable to walk a straight line. Mom tried to get ahead of him, but he threw his arm up and swung backward. Had Mom not ducked, he probably would have knocked her down.

"Let me drive, Junior. You're too drunk," she told him.

"I only had a couple. I'm fine."

"No, you're not. Look at you. You can hardly stand without falling. How do you think you can drive?"

She tried again to get between him and the driver's seat, but he pushed her away.

"Get in the car, or I'll leave you here."

I was ready to jump out and stay behind with Mom, but she finally slipped into the front passenger seat.

Dad opened the car door and got in behind the wheel. With him came the stench of stale cigarette smoke and beer. He fumbled with the keys until he finally found the ignition.

I heard my heart pound above the sound of the engine.

CHAPTER 2

THE UNLIKELY SHOWDOWN

The ride home proved to be worse than waiting in the alley. Dad refused to believe he wasn't sober enough to drive. Though the road had a few hills and dips, it ran straight—which wasn't how our ride went, as Dad weaved from one side of the road to the other. Somehow, he always made it back to the southbound lane before having a head-on collision with other cars. That fear was bad enough, but not as terrifying as the unforgiving bridge across Big Creek. I always held my breath until we crossed it, remembering news about a car that missed the bridge and landed upside down in the creek, killing the driver. I don't know how I thought digging my fingernails into the back of Mom's seat would save me, but I gave it my best effort.

Once we pulled in our driveway, I fell back against the seat with a sigh. The first terror had passed. I wondered what waited for us in the house. Dad's anger for getting pressed to leave the bar piqued.

"When's dinner going to be ready," Dad's question came out more like a demand.

"I don't know. What do you want? It's late to try to fix something. Do you want leftovers?"

"No. I don't want any *#^% leftovers." Dad's way of talking changed with the more beer he drank. It got loud, angry, and full of cursing, unless company was around.

I tried to stay out of his way—in another room, if possible—because he was in the mood to take his anger out on someone. I was his usual, easy target.

Why can't you just stay sober? That was my daily, silent plea. When he was sober, he never spanked me. But with each beer he consumed, the chances of my being whipped increased. And with Dad's drinking getting worse each year, the list of my infractions that resulted in a whipping expanded to things like not eating whatever was placed before me, especially vegetables that my tastebuds couldn't stomach, such as peas or butterbeans or spinach.

While Mom worked to get some meat and vegetables cooked and on the table, Dad fell asleep in his chair. Mom gave up trying to wake him. Mom, Kenny, and I sat to eat. I was thankful we had made it safely through another night.

Later that winter, we had a good snow. As a five-year-old, I loved it. It changed our yard into a new playground. In southern Illinois, where we lived, we could get all the way through winter with no snow. But this snow did more than cover the grass. It was deep and packed well, so Kenny took me out to build snowmen in the backyard. Afterward, he dragged out our sled. Our farm had no good hills for sledding, and our yard lay nearly flat as a table.

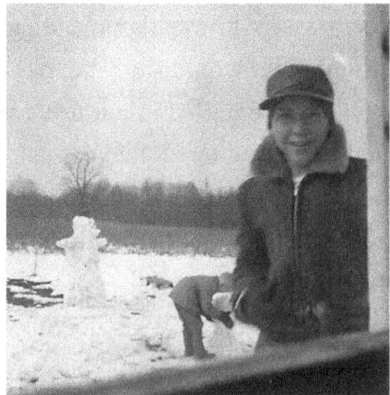

I am sort of in the picture bent over my snowman behind my brother.

"Sit down. I'll pull you around," Kenny told me.

Thrilled that he wanted to keep playing with me, I quickly obeyed. He grabbed the rope and pulled me around the yard. Although it didn't have the thrill of a hill, I enjoyed it.

"My turn," he said after a while. "You pull me." When he sat on the sled, it sank deep into the snow.

I took the rope and gave a tug. It didn't budge. I dug my heels in and leaned back, pushing with my legs as hard as I could. Nothing.

Kenny turned around and lay on his back on the sled, pushing with his feet as I pulled. Disgusted, he jumped up and headed for the house. "Well, that's no fun."

Mom had a surprise for us when I joined him inside. The deep snow made it good for snow ice cream. It tasted different from the home-made ice cream we cranked at family gatherings, but I liked it as much.

As I spooned in a taste, I got to thinking about Christmas, which was just around the corner. "Mom, how does Santa get into our house when we don't have a fireplace?"

"He still comes down the chimney."

"We should turn the furnace off then."

Mom said nothing.

"Don't you think we should?"

Still Mom said nothing, so Kenny jumped into the conversation.

"I'll show you. It's downstairs." With an air of confidence, he led me down the basement stairs where the chimney stood near the coal furnace.

For a moment I was afraid he would confirm that Santa crawls out of the furnace. I knew how hot that thing could get.

Instead, he pointed to a damper on the heater exhaust pipe. "Santa uses his magic to shrink himself and all the toys to come out that damper and carry the gifts upstairs where it all returns to normal size."

I checked on the status of the damper the next few days, not sure I believed Kenny's explanation, but I couldn't imagine a better solution. Christmas catalogs soon arrived in the mail, and their distraction helped me forget the how-does-he-do-it riddle. Looking through the toy pages united me with every other child in America. My deformities separated me from some activities, but not the excitement and anticipation of Christmas.

"Mom, when are we going to get our tree?"

"Christmas is still weeks away. If we get it too soon, it will dry out. It could become a risk of fire. We'll get it in time. Don't worry."

I checked off the days on the calendar, constantly reminding Mom how close Christmas was. Mom spent days after Thanksgiving making different candies: divinity, peanut brittle, fudge, date nut log, gradually setting some out the closer we got to Christmas. Her traditional holiday candy dishes, filled to the top, sat prominently on the coffee table and end tables in the living room—every candy she had made except those that needed to be refrigerated.

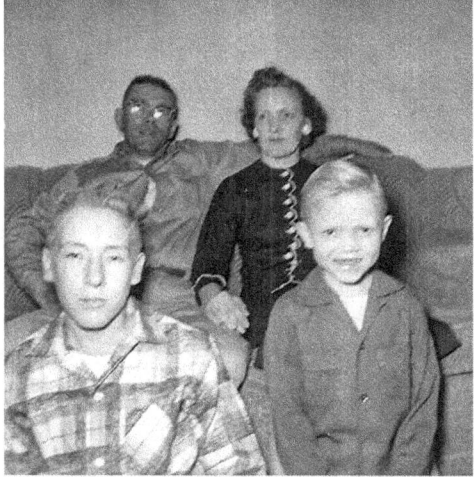
This is the only family photo I have: Dad, Mom, Kenny, and me.

When she pulled out the boxes of Christmas decorations, I knew getting the tree would be next. "Are you ready to pick out a tree?" she asked in a tone that suggested as much anticipation as I had swelling in me.

"Finally!"

With Dad at work and Kenny opting to stay home, Mom and I got in the car to drive to her uncle's farm in Iuka, about fourteen miles away. My anticipation made it seem like a much longer ride, but pulling into his driveway, I could hardly wait for the car to stop before jumping out to examine our next tree—any size for a dollar.

Arriving home with it, Kenny and Mom put it into the stand and filled the branches with the old familiar lights. Mom let me help hang the ornaments, completing the masterpiece by tossing bunches of aluminum silver tinsel on the tips of the branches until it looked like a snow-laden tree from outside. It transformed our living room, our home, into a magically happy place in my mind. I loved Christmas.

The holiday marked the time of year when evil seemed held at bay, while love for others had its moment in the spotlight. Even without the miracle I longed for, Christmas held an entrenched hope through the television specials with messages of peace and good will on earth. Besides the classic Christmas movies like *A Christmas Carol, A Miracle on 34th Street*, and *White Christmas*, regular programs had their own Christmas stories woven into their characters' lives. Even the thriller series *Twilight Zone* shifted its regular tone from bizarre morbidity to inexplicable occurrences of hope.

The old movie classics stirred a thought in me that maybe I was born in the wrong era, because I loved watching the men doff their hats while greeting neighbors on snow-covered streets. The respect shown one another. The disdain for immodest behavior. The intolerance toward public drunkenness and abusiveness. These all called out to me.

In my early years, Dad stayed sober on Christmas—partly because the taverns were closed. Blue laws in effect then required bars closed on Sundays and holidays. They gave me glimpses of the man Dad could be. I pretended that the man I saw those days was my everyday dad and the monster dad didn't exist. If only my dream world would last at least an entire day.

Removal of the blue laws changed that, and our weekly calendar oasis for us dried up. I awoke one morning to find our beautifully decorated Christmas tree less than perfect as it had been when I went to bed. It stood crooked, off balance. Decorations were no longer spaced out, and the tinsel was missing in some spots and overloaded in others.

"Mom, what happened to the tree?"

"Your dad. He woke me up cussing at someone to get out of his way so he could go to the bathroom. He was swiping at the tree, trying to knock it to one side or the other, convinced the bathroom was right behind it. He didn't want my help, but I finally got him turned around and into the bathroom."

One Christmas when I was seven or eight years old, Dad surprised us, or maybe especially me. Under the tree, my brother and I found the board game Monopoly. After we had unwrapped the presents and cleared away the debris, Dad opened the Monopoly game and set it up. I wasn't sure I wanted to play with Dad. He already had enough beer in him to slur his speech. I didn't know how long a fuse he might have. Plus, I never knew Dad willing to play anything that wasn't cards.

"Sit down and let's play!" he told Kenny and me.

I looked at Mom.

She smiled. "Go on. Give it a try."

I don't remember who won the game. I only recall having fun with my brother and Dad.

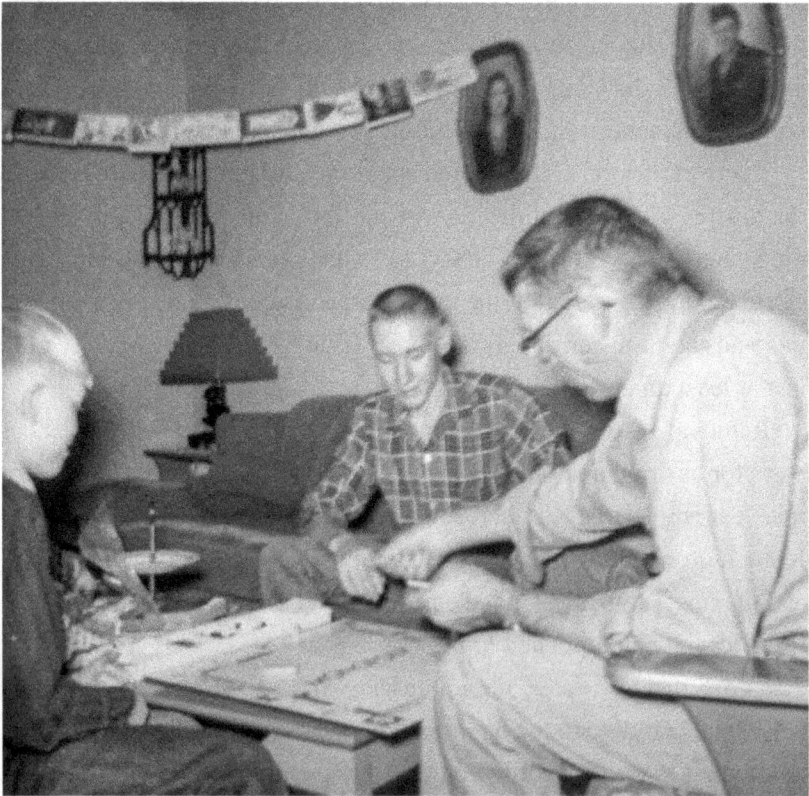

Until I was old enough to join the Pinochle games, this was the only bonding time I had with Dad.

Unlike the time when I was in Dad's arms, Mom took a picture of Dad playing with us. In spite of the fact that Dad had drunk too many beers before the game, and even though the picture Mom took of that moment never was displayed with honor in the family album, it occupied a special place in my heart.

I longed for that kind of Christmas miracle for the rest of time. But it didn't come. Eleven months of the year I hoped the next Christmas would bring on its tail a change in Dad. In time, not even the love of Christmas could keep him sober. Evil Dad settled in on my annual all-is-good holiday.

For the rest of the year, school served as another avenue of escape. The routine, the rewards for fulfilling expectations, even the rules that squeezed us into model behavior worked in my favor. While I was at school for a few hours each day, I could forget what was at home.

After Christmas break, we kids would compare what we each got. A couple of friends and I received hand puppets for Christmas, besides some other things, and decided we should put on a puppet show for the class. The teacher let us script it and practice it. She even created a simple stage for us. The class told us how much they enjoyed it. Yes, school was a safe place for me.

Friendships I developed there fed my need for diversion and, oddly, stability. I considered my friends being like family. I thought they would always be there—both with me and for me if I needed someone. A couple of years passed, and I learned how unrealistic that was. When my friends' parents took jobs out of the area or received a transfer, I lost more than a buddy. Not everyone in my class had the same connection with me. I looked at the remaining classmates and wondered who, if any of them, would be willing to know me better. Losing the one left a great, lonely ache. I tried to fill the void with another friend, but even replacements on my best-friends list ended up leaving.

The last one hurt the most.

Denny arrived at Grandma's, and after our customary joke exchange, I asked him about the unseasonal family get-together. "It's neat we are having a family gathering at Grandma's. Does anyone know why?"

Denny didn't hesitate with his answer. "Dad is being transferred with his job. We're moving to Oklahoma."

I considered Denny my closest cousin. Besides being only months younger than I, we liked many of the same things, especially using our wit and humor. Every time we were together, we competed to see who could make the other laugh more. We even talked about growing up to form a comedy team like Laurel and Hardy or Abbott and Costello. That dream blew up with his announcement. I wondered if he and our closeness would go the same way as the rest of my friends who left me.

He reassured me they planned on coming home every year on vacation to be here for the family reunions. That promise brought some comfort, but we dropped the subject to make the best of our last time together until who knew when. Not long after, they packed and moved.

Life continued for the four of us. Dad sometimes gone on trips, Mom always working on something. Kenny studied his high school courses, while my education had only begun. If not before, this marked the time I had become the annoying little brother Kenny dreaded I would be. Confident I had more abilities than my years, I nagged him to take me with him on his trips out of the house. Within his level of patience, he tried, like when he surprised me with, "Do you want to learn how to hunt mushrooms?"

It was early spring. The ground had thawed, but forest flowers hadn't bloomed. Morel mushrooms have a short growing season, so knowing the right time and the right places are essential for successful hunting. Before we reached the woods, Kenny started his instructions.

"Pay close attention to the ground around fallen trees and in low areas where the ground is still damp."

I nodded. It sounded simple enough.

"Also, they may be on the decaying tree trunks or pushing up under leaves."

I knew what the mushrooms looked like. I'd seen Mom wash, slice, salt, rinse, and cook them many times. What could be so hard?

I stayed close to him, waiting for him to lead me to what amounted to an adult-Easter-egg hunt. He stopped in one area and picked a few. I scanned the area but saw nothing. Like a magician pulling a quarter from an ear, Kenny reached into the forest floor and pulled out mushrooms. He made it look so easy.

"You have to look."

"I am looking." After that, I looked left and right as I followed behind him. The sharp tone of his last reminder tipped me off that I had done something wrong. All I saw was a giant collage of last fall's leaves.

A few times as he led me through fertile ground, Kenny reminded me of what he had told me. I was so excited when I found some that I couldn't wait to show him. Plus, I didn't want to irritate him by trying his patience by taking too long in one spot.

We were on our way out of the woods when he yelled at me for all the mushrooms we had left behind.

"We did? I didn't see any!"

"I told you and showed you how to find them. Each time I told you to be watching, we were passing by some. I left them for you to pick." He railed that we would have had more than twice the mushrooms if I had been looking. Our meager harvest was all my fault.

But it wasn't my fault. I was looking; I just didn't see them. I don't know why. He continued to beat me up with his words for a couple of minutes. He then stomped the rest of the way home in silence. At least his beating was with words only and not a belt.

As spring inched toward summer, I tried to fall in love with fishing to spend more time with him. It proved to be worse than hunting mushrooms. First, I couldn't keep up with him as we walked to neighbors' ponds, taking shortcuts through patches of woods and tall grass. Then I couldn't master the use of the reel, so the line kept tangling. I didn't bait the hook right. The bobber or the weights were too close to the hook. I jerked the line too hard and didn't set the hook, so the fish got away. Or I let the fish swallow the hook and made it hard to get out. That required interrupting Kenny for more help. He got little fishing done that day, and it was my fault again.

I don't know if it applied to people in general or just me, but Kenny rarely gave second chances. After the mushroom hunting failure, he never invited me along again. Considerable time passed after the fishing trip before he asked me to go with him anywhere. I jumped at his next invitation, although baffled by it as well. Too late for mushrooms, no fishing gear, no gear of any kind. We were just two brothers walking off into the woods. This trip went as near perfect as I could ever have hoped for. Like Dad, Kenny could sometimes be great to have around. This day he taught me something I treasured. Something I hated outgrowing. In a thatch of young trees, he pointed at one spindly sprout and told me to climb it until he said stop. "Now hold tight to the trunk with your hands and throw your legs out to the side."

This sounds dangerous. What if it doesn't bend as low as I need it to? I could break something or at the very least twist my ankle when I drop the rest of the way to the ground.

My fear of falling almost talked me into climbing down, but I remembered the fun Kenny and I had jumping off the corner of the garage roof onto a pile of hay. Afraid at first, I was so glad I took that chance.

I tightened my grip on the trunk and kicked against it with my feet so my body shot out to the side. As I did, the tree bent from my weight, lowering me back to earth. What a feeling! That ride was about as good as any ride in the carnival that came to town every year.

Kenny picked out a larger sapling for himself and joined in on the fun.

He taught me how to pick the right trees. "Too small of a trunk and you will drop too quickly. Too large and it will not bend."

When we quit, some young trees stood stooped over from the many rides. That day came to mind in my high school English class as we read Robert Frost's poem "Birches."

When I see birches bend to left and right
Across the lines of straighter darker trees,
I like to think some boy's been swinging them.

Before leaving the woods as we headed back home, we caught some small tree lizards. When we got to the house, we found the back door locked and Mom standing inside looking out at us.

"When you empty your pockets of what you found in the woods, I'll unlock the door for you."

How she knew, I could never figure out, but we gave up and let our new friends scamper away in the yard. Later, Kenny sneaked up behind Mom and brushed her neck with the tip of his finger. She jumped and spun around with a shriek, convinced we had slipped one last vermin in.

Even when we were relaxing around the television, Mom tried to be productive. Seeing her crocheting a new doily during one of the shows she enjoyed came as nothing unusual for me. Perhaps the oddest part of one evening was Dad's congenial mood. That day he had come straight home from work and had drunk only a few beers from his stock.

Kenny had left to be with friends. I lay on the couch. Dad lounged in his rocker and Mom sat in the overstuffed chair beside him.

During a commercial, I looked over at Mom. Her head lay back against the chair, and her arms hung loosely by her side. Something was wrong. "Mom!"

Dad noticed the alarm in my voice and followed my gaze toward her. He leaped from his rocker to reach her side. He lifted her head, patted her cheek. "Norma. Norma, talk to me."

Mom let out a little moan and pushed herself up with her elbows. She took hold of the crochet needle and began working it up and down, back and forth until she extracted it from the palm of her left hand. Somehow, she had impaled it. In trying to pull it out, it had snagged a tendon and caused her to faint.

Dad went with her to the bathroom to help clean and dress her wound. He showed once again he could be a man of the hour full of compassion and meeting the needs of another. I didn't want more trauma, but I did want to see more of that part of him.

I got my chance at that on the fourth Sunday of August with no crisis involved. Mom and Dad were working together to prepare their contribution to the family reunion potluck. Mom stood at the sink with her paring knife in hand, scraping the skin and pulling pinfeathers from a chicken for her family-famous fried chicken dish. Dad had a pot of potatoes boiling while chopping bell peppers, onions, and sweet dill pickles for the potato salad.

"Dad, are you fixing Mom's potato salad?"

"What makes you think it's Mom's?"

"I didn't know you knew how to cook."

"My last assignment in the army was mess sergeant. Yes, I know how to cook."

Our annual family reunions provided me with a safety zone. While at the family gatherings, Dad didn't drink. Other times, Dad managed—even when drunk—to be on his best behavior around other people. We saw the angry, violence-prone drunk, but around everyone else, he showed his congenial side. He rarely raised his voice around them. He might have given me a look of irritation now and then, but overall, he portrayed the appearance that all was good in the family. The good-guy image shattered as soon as we were alone again.

Those family gatherings boxed Dad into the image he wanted others to see of him. While the reunion lasted only a weekend, some family members often took vacation time and stayed in the area for a week. Those prolonged visits offered Mom and me the longest stretch of peace in our house in the year. By now, Kenny stood as tall as Dad, or maybe even a little taller. With high school graduation nearing, Kenny was often scarce around the house. If he wasn't with friends, he was out in the woods or at ponds and lakes fishing. Dad seemed to respect the man my brother was becoming and didn't try his authority over him, at last not physically.

The family reunion weekend delighted me almost as much as Christmas. I looked forward to the time with my cousins. True to his prediction, Denny and his family made it back to our hometown. We spent much of the weekend at Grandma's house or Uncle Bob's house. Both had large yards for us kids to romp in while the grownups sat and talked. I always heard a lot of laughter coming from their circle.

Usually Saturday night before the reunion gathering, those of us who had ice cream makers brought them to where we were getting together. The ladies mixed the cream while the men set the makers, rock salt, and blankets in the ready to crank the handles. When the ice cream became stiff, we kids took turns sitting on the maker to help steady it until the men could no longer crank it. Then they covered it with more blankets and allowed each one to freeze a few more minutes. Then heaven. Even the best ice cream on the market could not compare to what we made from scratch.

Sunday noon, Grandma Huff's brothers and sisters with their children and grandchildren came together with her tribe at a pavilion in the city park. Often we had more than one hundred family members attend. Upon arriving at the park, the adults busied themselves setting up the picnic tables for our potluck. The kids heard the annual rule to stay close to the pavilion until after lunch when we would then have full run of the park. After lunch, the adults held a business meeting that included recording updates on births and deaths in the family during the past year, election of new reunion officers, and entertainment.

With the festivity over, our branch of the family retreated to Grandma's house for a last hurrah until those who had to start back home said their goodbyes. Unless a cousin or two went home with me, by the end of the day, we would be again alone with Dad. I don't know if I let my imagination cloud the mood in the car as we pulled away from Grandma's, or if there had been a definite shift. I sat back in the seat with nothing to say. About halfway home, I had my answer.

"After I drop you off, I'm going back into town to meet up with Keith at the tavern," Dad said.

Mom fixed her eyes on him. "How long will you be gone?"

"Why? You have someplace you're planning on going?"

"No, of course not. I didn't know if you expected me to have supper for you when you got home and when that would be."

"I'm just going to have a couple of drinks with him, that's all."

With or without Uncle Keith, Dad never had just a couple of drinks. Maybe a couple he remembered, then the rest were lost. All I knew was Dad had held in his evil self long enough. And by the time Dad would return from the tavern, my happy time would come to a rapid end.

I arranged with a cousin or two to spend a night at our house later that week before they had to travel back home. I wondered what their homes were like when no one else was around. Did they have the same struggles with their dads? Then I thought about the television shows we liked to watch and how they portrayed family life. Television sons could go to their dads for advice. Their dads helped them navigate through the relationships at school, understand actions of others, try out a new skill, and be comfortable with who they are. But that was fiction. I could never go to my dad that way.

I did my best instead to stay out of sight and out of mind, which was nearly impossible in a house with only four small rooms. Dinners and television brought us together most nights—together as in proximity, not harmony. I turned on programs I knew Dad would enjoy, like *Gunsmoke, Maverick,* or *The Rifleman.* I was glad when he liked the same comedy shows I liked, such as *Ozzie and Harriet, Leave It to Beaver,* or *The Garry Moore Show.*

To keep the peace, I also learned to tolerate cooked carrots, hominy, and some other food items I had rejected before. Mom often played shortstop for me by saying in advance I didn't have to eat certain things so Dad wouldn't get mad.

As I grew older, I noticed that the whippings became fewer. Even so, there were days I didn't want to go to school for fear someone would somehow see my blue and purple stripes. I told no one about them. Shame held my tongue. Not a self-loathing shame—I knew I didn't deserve them. I simply didn't want anyone to know about Dad.

My heart ached to know what could change things for us. I had seen on television people praying for God to intervene for them and their situations. I knew nothing about God. In fact, I don't remember God's name spoken in our house unless Dad used it when cursing.

After another viewing of *It's a Wonderful Life*, I tried praying. I knew what I wanted most for Christmas was something I couldn't ask Santa for. "God, change Dad into a nice dad."

Is there a God? I wondered. *I guess there must be. Does He hear and answer our prayers?*

Nobody had ever told me anything about Him, until our first-grade class took a field trip to an afternoon matinee showing the newest Cecil B. DeMille's movie *The Ten Commandments*. I sat spellbound. When the Red Sea parted, I determined I would find out what I could about this God. Perhaps He was the answer I needed.

During recess at school the next day, I asked some of my classmates if they knew who God was. They knew only that He had many names: God, Father, Lord, Jesus, Christ, or Jesus Christ. They were no help. I decided to ask Mom. Since we had never talked about it, I didn't expect her to have answers, either.

"Well, God created earth and everything on the earth and in the sky. He had a Son, Jesus. It's His birth we actually celebrate at Christmas. Why do you ask?"

"You remember our class saw that movie? I want to know that God. I thought maybe He might help Dad. How does anyone get to know God?"

"You have to believe and be baptized."

"Wait. What's baptized?"

"You step into a tank of water. The pastor lays you down into the water, then stands you back up."

Water. I had three big fears: falling, darkness, and water. "Are you sure about that? I would have to be baptized? There's no other way?"

"I'm pretty sure."

Mom shared with me what she knew, and it was enough to stop my search for a while. The respect for God in her voice let me know why she had never used profanity, though it didn't explain why we had never talked about Him before. In all her childhood stories, she never mentioned Jesus.

A couple years later, Mom heard about a revival at a church in the area and asked if I wanted to go while Dad was out of town. The church had brought in an evangelistic team. Cecil Todd gave the message each night after Lowell Mason, the song evangelist, led the congregational singing and sang a special solo. Though considered a dwarf, standing at less than four feet tall (shorter than I was), Lowell's voice towered over everyone. He had an unbelievable range and his conversation oozed tenderness and love.

I asked Mom if we could go again. We ended up going every night. Early in the week, Cecil closed his message by telling about a nine-year-old girl who gave her heart to Jesus. He got my attention, because in about three weeks I would turn nine.

"She didn't know how her father would react," Cecil said. "He had never talked about God and church. He was always drunk."

Now I put myself into the story. The similarities were too strong not to.

"When the girl got home, her father asked where she had been all this time. She told him she had been to a special meeting at church where a minister told her wonderful things about Jesus. She added she had asked Jesus to come into her heart, and she had gotten baptized."

I sat up a little straighter.

"He jumped from his chair and whipped off his belt. He hit her with it over and over, ignoring her cries to stop. His rage never abated until his little girl lay before him bloody and dead."

I'm sure Todd had a good point to make with the story, but it slipped past me. I feared it could be my story, too, if I followed the prompting of my heart.

Each night I listened as Cecil and Lowell told about the great love of Jesus and the suffering he endured that we might have eternal life. Near the end of the evangelistic crusade, Cecil ended his sermon with a simple question, "Do you believe Jesus is the Son of God and that He died on the cross for you?"

By then, Mom and I had had more than a few conversations about God and His love. I believed she believed so I should too.

Cecil had convinced me of the truth of it. "If you believe, come down to the front here where we can pray with you."

I had been sitting with some new friends and not with Mom, so I had no one to hold me back or ask what I was doing. I could not push away the tug on my heart any longer. I simply stood and made my way toward the front with the others who were walking down the aisles. Not even the fear triggered by the girl's story from a few nights before could hold me back.

After a final call to anyone who might want to come forward to express their trust in Jesus Christ, Cecil said a prayer over us. We were all then led back to a room behind the podium where they asked questions and told us what we could do next. I listened as, one by one, those who came down to receive Jesus had an excuse for not getting baptized right then. Wanted to talk to parents first, wanted to be baptized in a different church, wasn't sure they were ready. Mom and I had talked already. The only thing that stood in my way was the water. I felt a reverse peer pressure. The more they excused themselves, the more I felt I had to complete what I had started.

I took my place in line to be baptized with two other remaining responders. As my turn came, I stepped into the water and sensed a peace blanket me. Placing my hand over my nose as instructed, I relaxed for the pastor to dip me. I came out of the water feeling like Jesus had wrapped Himself around me, shielding me, and protecting me in the water and back up again.

On the ride home, Mom looked at me curiously. "Why did you go down to be baptized?"

"I didn't really think I was going down the aisle for that. Cecil said for all who believed to come down and be prayed for. We've talked about this so, since I believed, I went down. Why didn't you?"

"I didn't know what to do. I was shocked when I saw you walking down. I probably would have stopped you had I been close to you."

"I'm glad I did, Mom. And Jesus protected me in the water."

The next day, Saturday, the evangelist and the local pastor Gerald came to our house to talk with Mom and Kenny. Dad was not around. All of this—the evening meetings, the meeting at our house, even the coming Sunday service—happened when he was on a long cross-country trip to deliver propane tanks. After listening to Cecil and the church pastor, Mom and Kenny prayed with the men and agreed to attend church the next day.

At Cecil's invitation at the end of his sermon that Sunday, Mom and Kenny walked forward and were also baptized. The church gave us baptismal certificates and pocket-sized versions of the book of John.

When we got home, Mom told us to hide our certificates. She put my certificate under a dresser drawer. Sometime later, Dad discovered my copy of the Gospel of John, accidentally left on an end table in the living room. He asked Mom where it had come from. She told him about the revival, our getting baptized, and receiving the certificates and gifts.

Dad's face turned scarlet. "Give them to me!"

Mom and Kenny retrieved theirs from where they were hidden and handed them to him.

"Outside now!" Dad grabbed a sack of garbage as he led the way. He threw the sack into our burn barrel and lit it. Then he threw the little Gospels along with Mom and Kenny's baptismal certificates into the fire. "I'll not have this in my house. Did you get anything else?"

If I weren't so afraid, I would have been crying.

Dad fixed his glare on me. "Where's your certificate? Give it to me."

"I don't want to."

"I don't care what you want. I said give it to me."

"No. Please."

Dad started unbuckling his belt. I wondered if the others could see how much my body was shaking. *Looks like I'll soon know firsthand the rest of that girl's story.* Before Dad slipped his belt out, I lost sight of him. Kenny now stood between us.

"He said he doesn't want to. Leave him alone."

"I'll whip you, too. Don't think I won't."

"I doubt it. Besides, burning that won't change a thing."

Dad glared at him. He took a step toward Kenny, but Kenny didn't flinch. They locked eyes in a stare down.

I held my breath. I had never seen anyone oppose Dad in such a way. Would Kenny be able to win a fight against him? Most incredible to me was Kenny confronted Dad for my sake. He was willing to go to blows if it came to that for me.

My lungs started to burn. Dad broke the stare contest and went back into the house. I started breathing again. The crisis passed for the moment.

The next day I went to the burn barrel to look through the ashes. I found what I thought was my copy of John's Gospel. I looked wide-eyed as I flipped through the pages, scorched on one corner but with not one word missing. "Are you trying to tell me something, God?"

Dad tried one more time to destroy the hope I held onto in sheer desperation. About a week later, he came home late from the bar. Kenny and I were already in bed and nearly asleep when he staggered into our bedroom and ordered me out of bed. Kenny jumped up and invaded Dad's private space.

"I told you to leave him alone. I'm trying to sleep. Now get out of our bedroom."

Again, Dad retreated. He knew he could out-wait Kenny. After all, Kenny, who was now nearly eighteen years old, had signed up for the navy, and would be leaving soon.

As Kenny got back into his bed and rolled over, I came to appreciate Kenny's new role in my life: protector. But it was ending too soon. Fear wrapped its tendrils around my heart and squeezed.

CHAPTER 3

THE MONSTER SPRANG

Three weeks after the revival, I turned ten. A few days later, Mom and I dropped Kenny off at the train station for Navy boot camp training. As I watched him board, my heart felt heavy. *My protector is gone. Nothing is at the house to hold Dad back from his rages.*

When Saturday evening came, Dad seemed in a good mood for a change. "If you want to go to church tomorrow, you can. I will drop you off and pick you up afterward."

I didn't know what to think about this sudden turn. He hated everything to do with Christianity. What changed his mind? Though I hoped this signaled a softening of his heart, I suspected some evil in his motives.

Although I never heard Grandma say much to Dad about Jesus, I instinctively knew Dad's mom prayed for him. She made comments when he wasn't around, most often when her neighbor would stop in to rehearse their duets for Sunday service. Maybe telling him she wished he didn't drink so much was all she had left to say. One of Dad's aunts stepped in where she left off, sending him notes of encouragement in the mail, sometimes throwing in a Scripture or two. She even bought him a Bible and sent it to him. Could her efforts to minister to him be paying off?

Maybe he won't just drive us, but actually go to the service with us. Maybe he'll consider it easier to sit with us in the service than driving us back and forth. I wanted to hold onto hope that this may be a real change in him.

But the next Sunday yielded no change. He drove us to church and waited at the curb when we came out. Every week was the same, although he complained if we took too long getting out.

I always sat quietly in the back seat and looked at that week's handouts and the new lesson booklet. I liked going to church. The pastor had two boys close to my age who took me under their wings, so to speak. We were becoming good friends. Mom even arranged for them to visit our house on some days when Dad was away on delivery trips.

Dad's delivery trips yielded other rewards. Arriving home from school one day, I called out, "I'm home."

"What do you think you'd like for dinner tonight?" Mom said.

"Why?"

"Your dad's gotten called out for a long haul. He won't be home tonight. Maybe not tomorrow night either."

"Pizza!"

I loved those nights when Dad wasn't going to be home because he was on the road. Those were the times when Mom and I could freely study our Sunday school lessons and read the previous Sunday's handouts together. She even bought herself a new Bible. I thought it was the grandest thing ever. It nearly replaced the family photo album as my go-to diversion. The topical reference section opened new portals to explore. The colorful pictures of several Bible stories helped bring the events to life.

It felt good to have bits of peace to enjoy. Even the weekly drives to church held little tension, since Dad had drunk no beers in the day, yet. But because he stocked up a supply for the weekends, we never knew what the ride home would be like until we got into the car after church.

One Sunday's drive home upended everything I thought I knew about Dad. He was sober, so the five miles home passed uneventful and pleasant. In fact, he seemed so fatherly that afternoon that I sat behind him instead of my normal safer distance behind Mom. As Dad started his turn into our drive, a frightful squall of tires pierced the air. I spun around to see a car jerk into the next lane, barely missing our rear bumper, but into the path of an oncoming car.

Dad whipped into our drive, skidding on the gravel. He stomped the brakes as soon as we were off the highway and jumped out. I sat breathless as the car that avoided us pulled back into the right lane, missing the oncoming car. I guess the driver lost control, because, instead of straightening out in the lane, the car continued its trajectory and drove off the road. Hitting the embankment on the opposite side of the drainage ditch, the car went airborne, flipped end over end and spun one complete rotation at the same time. It landed on its four wheels in our field, encased in a thick cloud, which suggested fire to me.

I didn't see my monster running toward it. I saw my dad. My fear *of* Dad shifted to a fear *for* him. I had never felt that before. "Stop, Dad! It might blow up!"

The cloud thinned as Dad reached the car and looked in. My heart still raced. Then I realized the cloud wasn't smoke from a fire. It was nothing more than dust. The car's impact had kicked up dirt from the field.

How did Dad know? Did he know? Would it have made a difference? With that crisis past, I ran to catch up with him.

The rear window had shattered in the crash. Through the opening I saw someone sitting in the rear passenger seat, slumped over the back of the front seat.

Dad opened the door to check on them. It was a woman, and Dad reached in to help her out. A tricycle entangled around her legs and wedged between the seats pinned her until Dad managed to remove it. She took Dad's hand and stood. He held her steady until she could stand unattended.

I watched Dad's face take on a look I'd not seen before. On another man, I would have called it fear. His eyes darted from the tricycle to the other toys in the car and to the missing rear glass. He then scanned the seats and floorboards, but he didn't see anyone. "Was anyone else with you?"

"No. I was alone. I was taking these toys to my son. My husband and I separated recently. I was headed down to give my boy some things for his birthday."

Dad relaxed. "Are you okay?"

"My back. I feel burning pain in my back."

Dad turned her around. A red stripe traced her spine down her blouse. Dad lifted it and began pulling out chunks of the rear windshield.

All the dust had settled by now, so I walked over to look inside the car. I couldn't figure out how she got from sitting behind the steering wheel to sitting in the backseat on the opposite side of the car.

Mom walked up to tell us she had called for an ambulance and the sheriff, both arriving a few minutes later.

The sheriff asked me what I knew about the accident. I told him I had been sitting right behind Dad, with my arms crossed on the back of his seat.

"Do you know if he signaled he was going to turn?"

"Yes, he did."

"Are you sure? This is very important."

"Yes. I remember seeing the little green arrow flashing on the dashboard and hearing the clicking noise."

He asked what happened next, so I told him all I had seen and heard. Satisfied, he turned and talked to the lady who was on a stretcher by then.

She told the sheriff she had looked away at the countryside and didn't see we were turning until she looked back at the road. "It was all my fault. I'm just glad I didn't hit anyone."

The sheriff took notes and asked what she wanted done with her car, then radioed in for a wrecker.

The response team left shortly thereafter. Only the scar on our field testified to the harrowing event we had been through. It also disappeared after a few days. One thing remained. Inside the monster I called Dad stood a brave man, a hero in my eyes, and I discovered I hadn't lost all my love for him.

That accident and its aftermath heralded something new between Dad and me. A few weeks into summer after the accident, he decided to reclaim some of our tillable land from the encroaching woods. Each year saplings grew into the fields, slowly expanding the woods and shrinking the fields. He assembled his arsenal of shovels, chain, Mom, me, and our tractor. We headed to a small grove of trees in the middle of one field. Mom and Dad always called that thicket the Old Home Place, since it was the site of my great-great-granduncle's log cabin.

Dad gave me instructions on the steps we would take and what my role would be. "Show me you can push in the clutch."

I did as he directed.

"Okay, good. When I say stop, I want you to push in the clutch as fast as you can."

Mom objected to having me on the tractor. "He's too young, Junior."

Dad wasted no time with getting ensnared in such a conversation. Instead, he dug around a young tree to loosen the dirt around the roots, wrapped the chain around the base of the trunk, and attached the other end of the chain to the tractor.

I sat at the wheel with the tractor in gear, throttle up, and my foot holding in the clutch—waiting. When Dad said, "Pull," I let up the clutch and pulled the sapling out. Dad yelled stop, and I pushed in the clutch and slipped the gearshift back to neutral. I did it.

I turned to see Dad happy with me, but nothing. No smile. No gesture to signal, *Good job*. Not even a glance in my direction. He was busy removing the chain from that sapling and going to the next.

Mom stood wide-eyed for a moment, then pulled the uprooted sapling out of the way. Then she went back to Dad. "I think he's too young. Remember how our neighbor's girl was crushed by the tractor she was on a few months ago? They were doing much the same thing, only she didn't get the clutch pushed in soon enough and the tractor lurched forward then tipped back on top of her."

Dad let on like he wasn't listening, so Mom persisted. "We should get someone else to help you. The clutch is tight and hard for him to push."

Her arguments had no effect on Dad, but she succeeded in putting a healthy fear into me. In spite of that and because of the inner desire to please Dad, I claimed my place and right to be there. "I know how to do this, Mom. I'll be okay."

Dad's determination pushed us onward. Several more saplings yielded to me and the tractor with little or no fight. All went according to plans until one sapling had stronger or deeper roots. I felt the front wheels lift off the ground and immediately pushed in the clutch. Mom screamed. The wheels banged back to earth. Dad shut the tractor off.

That ended my farming experiences with Dad. He sold the tractor and rented out the fields. With farming duties completely gone, the house became little more than his place to sleep off his drunken state. Dad had nothing at home demanding his time and attention. Nothing except Mom and me.

He started volunteering for the longer cross-country hauls, which created a different problem for him. His long-haul trips delivering tanks became an inconvenience for him when Mom needed the car while he was gone. That called for us having to pick him up from work, and he didn't always get back to the shop at quitting time. Plus, he didn't like being nagged to leave the tavern before he was ready. He bought a second car for Mom. It was much older than the used car he drove, but it got us to town and back for laundry, groceries, or any other errands. Plus, we could drive ourselves to church. The greatest advantage for me was no more terror-filled rides home with Dad at the wheel. People talk about teens approaching life as if they will never die. I, on the other hand, wondered if I would even see my teen years.

Mom driving us to church settled well with Dad, because it meant he could either stay home and drink or go to the taverns that were now open on Sundays. Safe days with sober Dad became fewer.

Late one evening that fall, Dad came home late, drunk and angry, and my worst fears morphed into reality. Mom stood at the bathroom sink doing her bedtime ritual of brushing her hair, washing her face, and brushing her teeth. I had not gotten ready for bed when I thought of a question to ask Mom. From the hallway, I saw Dad reach into the gun cabinet that stood near the front door. My heart raced as I watched Dad lift out his pump shotgun, fumble for some shells, and begin loading them into the clip.

I squeezed close to Mom. *It's too dark for hunting. That limits his target to someone in town who angered him . . . or us.* "What's Dad doing with his gun?"

"I don't know." Mom dried her hands and tossed down the towel, then brushed past me to get to Dad. She grabbed the gun and tried wrestling it away from Dad. His imbalance from too much to drink worked in her favor, but his strength compensated for a tense struggle.

I noticed he was standing on the end of a floor runner. They always slipped easily on Mom's well-waxed wood floors. *Maybe I can pull the rug out from under him so he'll fall.* But I realized that wouldn't work. *I might not have the strength against his size, and I would just make him angrier. Or maybe he would fall on Mom.*

While I argued with myself about what to do, I doubted my ability to help in any way. Dad had so much size and strength advantage over my nine-year-old body and strength. As I stood behind Dad, I froze.

If only Kenny the Protector had still been here, none of this would be happening. Kenny had the size and strength to stand up against him. *What if I got on my hands and knees so Mom could push Dad and make him fall over me?*

In my mental frenzy, I didn't see how Mom broke Dad's grip on the gun. I only saw her throw it across the room, and Dad turn to retrieve it. Mom opened the front door and said, "Let's go!" I followed Mom out, and as I did so, I turned the lock button on the door.

I imagined Dad grabbing the doorknob and giving it a yank. Maybe he was drunk enough that its resistance confused him, made him lose his grip. He would have to unlock the door before it responded to him. How much time would that buy us? A second? Maybe as much as fifteen seconds, if we were lucky? We were desperate, and any amount would help.

Mom and I ran toward our neighbor's house across the highway. The open landscaping provided no place to hide. We jumped down into the ditch next to the road when we heard the front door of the house slam. Without a moon that night, darkness cloaked us. It no longer loomed as something for me to fear. Darkness was our friend. Without it, we would have been easy targets.

Our car's engine roared to life. *He's going to use the car's head-lights to remove our cover.* We watched the shadows form and move around as Dad maneuvered the car into position. We tried to sink deeper into the shadows of the ditch. Like the prison searchlights I had seen in the movies, the car lights swept the landscape, passing over where we lay.

I knew the next sound I'd hear would be the car door as Dad got out with his shotgun to finish his hunt. Instead, the car pulled out of the driveway, pointed toward town. Maybe he thought we were heading to his uncle's house and could catch up to us.

Or maybe this is a ruse to get us to come out of hiding. He is going to turn around and shine the lights in our eyes.

We peeked up the road, then sat up, watching while the taillights grew smaller and closer together. *He's going back to town.*

We got out of the ditch and ran to the neighbor's house, which sat far back from the highway. Tonight, their yard sprawled before us like a football field. Mom had bloodied her knees when she jumped into the ditch, so Bernice wet a washcloth and handed it to Mom along with some bandages. She and her husband grimaced and shook their heads as Mom explained what had happened.

They insisted we could not go back home. We had to find a safe place to live. They were so firm in their protection, they wouldn't let Mom go back to the house alone to pack some clothes. Instead they called the sheriff who came and accompanied Mom. She packed two suitcases in record time.

Dad had grabbed the keys to the other car before leaving, so Mom made a quick phone call to Dad's brother who lived nearby. He picked us up at our neighbor's house and gave us a ride to Mom's parents two hours away. My fears didn't leave; they only shifted.

I'll have to start a new school. What will it be like? Will I be able to make any friends? It won't take Dad any time at all to find where we've gone. Grandpa's would be the first place to look. What will he do when he finds us? Have we put Grandma and Grandpa in danger now too?

Grandma took us to a secondhand store where we bought some clothes to fill our wardrobe gaps. School was a short walking distance from their house, but it met my expectations. I didn't find it to be a friendly place. Each walk home would have been happier than the walk to school, except for my wondering if Dad would be there waiting for me.

Nearly a week went by before Dad found us. He called and talked with Mom. A few days later, he called again. And then again. I kept telling Mom I didn't want to go back.

The constant calls, the changes he promised, the uncertain future we faced, and maybe even Dad's past threats to kill her if she ever tried to leave wore Mom's resolve down.

"He said he has gotten rid of the guns."

"How? Where?"

"He didn't say. He only said he can't get his hands on them again. They're gone. He also said he has stopped drinking and even went to church with his mom last Sunday."

It sounded like everything I had prayed for, but this time the threat of death had gotten too close. I didn't want to take a chance. However, no amount of pleading on my part changed her mind. Dad picked us up that weekend and took us home.

The second car no longer sat in the driveway. Dad sold it first thing. Fear took a bite out of me. But I relaxed a little when I saw the empty gun cabinet. No beer in the refrigerator gave us more hope.

After work the next week, Dad stopped at the bar before coming home. He never went to church with us. Then, as hunting season rolled around the next fall, the guns reappeared in the cabinet.

CHAPTER 4

A SILENT BUT
SWELLING VOLCANO

Dad had told us the guns were where he couldn't get his hands on them again. No, he hadn't sold them, but he couldn't get them back. Yet there they sat in the gun cabinet as before. *Where had they been? Had someone been holding them for him? Why did they let him have them back?* These thoughts swirled in my mind as I kept watch over the gun cabinet, looking for the slightest change. Ten-year-olds are too young for such responsibility.

As more days and months passed without any changes in the cabinet, I relaxed my vigil. Nearly two years had passed since Dad loaded his shotgun that night. He had more days of being sober or at least only a few beers than being drunk. We almost resembled a family. Mom and I appreciated the reduction of aggression and learned to live with the tension. The beatings stopped, though the threats didn't. And Dad's ready access to the guns kept me in high alert, robbing me of sleep without fear. I never knew if I would see the sun rise.

Eventually Dad's drinking inched back up, cutting into the comfort spread of more good days than bad ones. We slipped back into the pattern of family reunion, pinochle nights, and Christmas serving as islands of refuge in our calendar. They gave me an escape from thinking about my family's secret battle. On those days, I could pretend

Mom, Dad, and I lived like I imagined the families of any other home in America—the ones I watched on television every night.

Yes, Dad was nothing like the fathers we saw on television, but Mom had her differences, too. Like the TV mothers, Mom was a peacemaker in the family. And she wore a dress around the house. However, it was her work-around-the-house dress, and she wore no makeup or jewelry. Not so with Harriet Nelson, June Cleaver, and Margaret Anderson.1 But also unlike them, Mom's house chores surpassed all they did. While they cooked and cleaned and shopped, their city lives demanded little else from them, compared to our country life. Except for running the rototiller, Mom's part in raising a garden included planting, weeding, hoeing, guarding against worms and other pests, and harvesting. Occasionally, Dad helped rototill.

Fresh produce from her garden enriched our table all summer. Several days found her sweating over the steaming pans while she canned or froze as much as she could. She stocked our shelves and freezer so we had plenty to eat through the winter.

Without Dad around, or not in any condition because of his drinking to do work at home, Mom used what she knew about carpentry to make modifications and repairs. She taught me how to paint. She sewed most of her clothes from bolts of material. She would have made mine, too, but I insisted on store-bought. She reupholstered and refinished furniture. If it weren't for her, our house would have reflected the shamble of Dad's life.

And to the limit of her ability, she protected me. She often used distraction to redirect Dad when she saw him reaching for his belt. And she never told him of things I did that deserved discipline. She much preferred handling the situation herself and leaving him out of it.

The dread of Dad's anger being unleashed again hung suspended above me like an executioner's axe. I finally got up the nerve to ask Mom, as we sat one day prepping green beans for canning, why we left our safe place with Grandma and Grandpa to return to Dad's unpredictability.

"I didn't think we could make it on our own. I didn't know what I could do for work. It's been such a long time since I've worked outside the home. If a place wanted someone with experience, I didn't have any."

Her answer didn't satisfy me, even though a part of me was glad we were back. I preferred our small hometown of about seven thousand people over the city life in Decatur. I loved our family reunions and being around neighbors I knew, which we couldn't do if we lived there.

I dropped the subject without asking her my real question: Would she have stayed with her parents if I wasn't around? I was a high-maintenance child needing special-order shoes. Every three months I had to keep hospital or clinic appointments. And sometime before I got too old, I would have foot surgeries scheduled for the last stage of correction.

If I were dead, would it make a difference? I would be free from Dad's threats. Mom might be able to leave and pursue the life she deserved. I was too chicken to consider harming myself, but it didn't stop me from wondering.

"Are you ready to help me get the jars, rings, and lids ready for canning?" Mom's question brought me back from my mental meanderings to the pans of snapped beans on the table.

"Can I?"

"First we need to scald the jars, rings, and lids." Mom set the pans of water on the stove to boil, then spread out towels to set the jars and lids to air-dry. "We have to finish these today so I can pick up Uncle Roy and Aunt Sarah's laundry tomorrow. We have a full day tomorrow."

I had forgotten about them. In addition to everything else she did, she helped Dad's aging two spinster aunts and another uncle and aunt of his. I realized Mom might have returned with Dad because of these other commitments. The selfless way she served taught me that love of others makes a house a home.

I opened the new box of lids and popped them apart as Mom instructed me, dropping them into the small pan of boiling water. I smiled as I thought of all Mom did for the good of others, yet still found time for rubber-band fights and other bits of fun with me, too. *She's a great mom*, I thought, a fun memory coming to mind.

Several years before, curiosity and boredom had sent me on an archeological excursion through Dad's dresser drawers while he was at work. I must have been nine-years-old, maybe, and had no idea what I hoped to find. I had convinced myself certain treasures lay hidden there. Slipping my hand under his briefs, socks, and handkerchiefs, and sliding my hand around the bottom of the drawer, I found a gold pocket watch, among other items. Mom later told me it was Dad's railroad watch. He got it when he worked on the railroad for a time. Interesting information; I never knew he had worked on the railroad.

But the most interesting discovery lay in a different drawer, also covered with clothes. I found a small stack of magazines Dad had picked up at truck stops on his cross-country deliveries.

I glanced through the magazines, and to my amazement, I saw pictures of naked people living in a nudist colony. Mom walked into the room just at that moment. I knew I was wrong going through their drawers, but I had taken the risk, feeling it would be worth it. Expecting a sharp reprimand, I saw in her face more embarrassment than anger with me. She closed the magazine I had open in my lap, picked up the small stack of magazines, and told me to follow her into the living room. This was totally not what I expected. What happened next surprised me even more. Retrieving two pairs of scissors, Mom sat down, picked up a magazine, and started to cut out selected pictures. She told me to do the same with the scissors she handed me.

At first, I sat befuddled. She then explained that we were going to pull a trick on Dad. When we clipped enough images for her prank, she then put the magazines back in his dresser drawer so he wouldn't suspect anything. Neither of us said anything about it when he got home. We had supper, watched some television, and went to bed.

While Dad was getting ready for work the next morning, Mom did her usual routine of fixing him breakfast and packing him a lunch. She needed the car for errands that day so she also got dressed to take him to work. The one thing she did different was to replace the meat in Dad's sandwiches with the pictures we had clipped. She added a tossed-picture salad for extra measure.

On the way to pick Dad up from work later, I giggled in the back seat, squirming in excitement to see how Dad received our joke. Mom looked in the rearview mirror at me. "Get your giggles out now before we get into town. You have to sit quiet like nothing has happened when your dad gets in the car. Okay?"

More giggles. "Okay."

Mom had gotten distracted from watching the time as she prepared things for cooking dinner. That made us late getting to Dad's workplace, so he was already standing outside the gate waiting. She maintained a straight face as if nothing were out of the ordinary. I somehow managed to do the same, or at least enough not to draw his attention. I noticed an odd expression as he slipped into the front passenger seat.

He turned to give Mom a stern look. I noticed a twinkle in his eye that betrayed him. "Think you're smart, don't you?"

"Why do you say that?" Mom looked questioningly at him.

"You know."

"No, I don't." Mom couldn't hold it any longer and started laughing.

Dad kept his eyes on her, and I guess he was enjoying her laughter because the twinkle in his eyes grew. I had seen that twinkle before. It was like the one he gave when he trumped his opponent's ace in Pinochle. "I just want you to know it backfired on you."

Now Mom was curious. "How so?"

"When you were late getting here, one guy said you were probably at the newsstand buying supper."

We laughed—a great, warm laugh. Dad had a sense of humor. We *could* have fun as a family. Without the alcohol, Dad could be like one of those television fathers. The happy spell over the family continued the rest of the night.

I blinked as I looked back down at the canning jars. We hadn't seen Dad that fun loving in a long time. Even our Pinochle nights carried a weight of tension now. Thankfully, most of it had to do with how the cards played out.

Mom sometimes sat in on a few hands, but mostly she found time and strength to be a good hostess. At least one Friday or Saturday night a month—often weekly, we had family or friends in to play pinochle. It held such a place in our lives and habits that it defined us. A person wasn't a Huff if he or she didn't play the game. I learned how to play in junior high. After years of watching others bid and play their hands, I got to join the grown-ups at the table. Dad had fewer beers those nights, so we enjoyed a level of family life.

The rest of the weeknights, Dad resumed his stopping for a beer after work. Mom hoped—we hoped—Dad meant what he said and would limit it to one drink while we waited in the car. Occasionally, Mom and I window-shopped to pass the time. Together, we sat until Dad later staggered out, again insisting he was sober enough to drive.

Dad's frequent rages, the threatening gun cabinet, and his erratic driving convinced me I could expect a short life. I hated that. I hated the alcohol that fueled it. Hatred toward Dad crept up to take a seat beside my fear of him. The gulf between us grew wider and deeper.

One morning after a game night, the phone rang and Dad answered it. His mother was on the other end. Having figured that out, I turned my focus back to the Saturday morning cartoons. When he hung up, Mom and Dad's conversation got my attention. Dad said his mom had started sorting through things to get rid of after holding onto everything for six years since Grandpa died.

"She wants me to come get the Japanese rifle out of her house. I can see if I can sell it."

I jumped into the conversation. "Japanese rifle? What Japanese rifle?"

Dad had talked very little about his experiences in World War II— even when I pushed him. This bit of information had never come up.

"After the war ended, the Japanese had to surrender their weapons. The rifles were stacked like thatches of wheat according to their condition. The best ones in piles only high-ranking officers could choose from on down through the ranks to the rifles in the worst condition for lowest ranks. The army let us take one of each item if we wanted until the last ones were taken."

"So you got a rifle?"

"With a bayonet and officer's sword."

"Don't sell them. I want them."

"Why? What would you do with them?"

"Keep them. I love antiques. They are a piece of history." I paused, then added, "They belonged to you." I think I added the last line because a part of me still wanted to honor and love the hero I'd glimpsed on rare occasions. Maybe they reminded me of the dad in the picture I lingered over. Or I could have thought flattery would get my way. Besides, that gun posed no threat since he said he had no bullets for it.

The discussion ended. A few days later, Dad brought the old weapons home from his mom's house. The sword caught my attention with its carved figures on the hilt lying under a thin leather black ribbon woven over them. I traced the images and strapping with my fingers. Unsheathing it revealed a long, heavy sword still very sharp. I put it back in its sheath and set it aside. The gun was heavier and had evidence of battle. I figured out how to attach and detach the bayonet. When I had finished, Dad put them in the gun cabinet.

A few weeks passed before a man came to the house and started talking with Dad about buying the gun. I had never seen this man before. He wasn't one of Dad's hunting, work, or drinking buddies I had met. I sat listening with a sickening heart, wondering how he knew about the gun. I guessed Dad's mind was made up to sell it. This was grown-up business, and Dad didn't like interruptions. I knew I didn't dare speak up, so I sat quietly, feeling worse by the minute. I half heard the man make an offer when Dad said, "You will have to talk with him." He gestured toward me with his thumb.

"Me?"

"You said you wanted it. It's yours. Do you want to sell it? It's a good price."

I couldn't say a word for a moment as I tried to make sense of what Dad just said. *Does the sale really depend on my say?* I looked at Dad and slowly shook my head. "No, I don't want to sell it."

The man changed his tactic. He had a German rifle he offered to trade with me. Dad must have seen my resolve weakening. In my mind, a German weapon connected with our ancestry, and it was still part of history and the war. But what about my comment to Dad? The gun we were haggling over held sentimental value because Dad had picked it for himself after the war. Before I answered, Dad told me I would never be able to shoot the German rifle around our parts. "It has a stronger kick. Its bullet travels farther. If you ever think you want to fire the gun, you should keep the one you have."

That settled it. That day I became the proud owner of a World War II Japanese rifle, bayonet, and officer's sword. Incredible. And best of all, it had belonged to my dad. He had given it to me. This marked the first time in twelve years he indicated he cared about my feelings. *Maybe he likes me after all.*

Another year passed. That included many more hazardous trips across the Crooked Creek bridge with drunken Dad behind the wheel. Each successful crossing left me wondering if I was living a charmed life. Maybe the God I was learning about at church was working in my life, though I couldn't be sure. Teachings at our church limited miracles to the wonders of birth, spring after the dead of winter, and other beautiful events in the natural world. The miracles in the Bible were nothing more than that—stories in the Bible and not happening these days.

For the previous two summers, Mom had signed me up to attend a week at the Oilbelt Christian youth camp. The missionaries who were guest speakers there had a very different message about the God who divided the Red Sea. One story they told gave me hope. The missionary had been with primitive African tribes who still lived as they did centuries earlier. He held our attention with his account of being dragged out of his hut in the middle of the night. The anger and force with which the tribesmen led him on his way triggered fear and questions. Had he done something to offend the tribal leader?

Making their way to his unknown destination, the men told him someone from their village had been attacked, and they wanted him to pray to his God for healing. The future of his work with this people and maybe his own life depended on what happened next. Entering the hut where the wounded man had been laid, he realized this situation needed a miracle. The man had been hit in the head with an axe. His skull was split open. His brain, swollen, pushed through the crack. The missionary moved to the end of the table where he lay and silently prayed as he applied pressure to squeeze the skull back together. He cried out aloud for the young man who was one of his first to understand and accept the gospel. He pleaded with God for that miracle. The next morning the young man walked around, fully healed.

Of the many stories the missionary told, none captured my attention more. I reminded God of that story many times as I pleaded for miracles in my life. Besides longing for the change in Dad, I had one other repeated petition. In my elementary to teen years, I was prone to coming down with tonsilitis. I'd get a fever, then my tonsils got sore, then my throat would nearly swell shut. The first sign I was getting sick was that I'd have a nightmare. It was the same scene every time. A mechanical monster chased me. Climbing stairs or even a ladder did not enable me to escape. It seemed able to reason and anticipate my defenses, strong enough to crash through locked doors. All this even though it moved on wheels instead of feet. It terrorized my sleep and my waking.

The summer between seventh and eighth grades, I had my first foot surgery, the final step toward correcting my club feet. Dad's drinking continued to worsen. Our car still staggered home and crossed the bridge. Mom and Dad still argued. And I still wondered why none of my miracles happened.

At least the mechanical monster in my nightmares stopped. In the hospital after surgery, I sat in the wheelchair with its arm that reached up to hold drip bags if necessary. It wasn't evil nor permanent. It had no hold on me. That monster died when I saw it for what it was.

Before the hospital sent me home, the doctor cut off the long-leg cast to replace it with one that reached from my foot to just below my knee. I saw the cuts made on my foot as they redressed the bandages. I looked for stitches all around the leg above the ankle for what I saw looked like an entirely new foot, not mine modified. The hump on my arch was gone along with the inward curve. I saw a narrow foot, straight—a normal foot. I refused to cry in front of the doctor.

After a few successful walks on crutches, I got to go home. Trying to tell Mom about the foot missed its mark on the impact intended. I almost face-planted the first time I navigated down the front stairs of our house. Thankfully, only one step sat between the porch and the sidewalk, which I flew past on my way down.

Getting in and out of the car remained difficult long after I mastered the stairs. One night we arrived home in the twilight hour between dusk and darkness. As I struggled to get out of the car with my plaster encased leg and crutches, Dad continued his argument with Mom. They had left me to get out and catch up to them as they headed for the back door. Then erect with the crutches positioned in my armpits, I looked up when Dad hit her.

I extended the tips of my crutches forward as far as I could and swung my body to the maximum reach, long-jumping to where Dad stood with his back toward me. As I came up behind Dad, I let go of one crutch and raised the other overhead to hammer down on Dad. I stopped. *Where should I hit him? How hard? I want to knock him out so he doesn't get back up swinging, but I don't want to kill him. What if I land the crutch in the wrong place?*

Angry-me spoke in my ear, "What does it matter. He deserves this. Hit him!"

Son-me countered. "He's your dad. You don't really want to hurt him like he's hurt you. Remember your prayers for him. Remember your love."

Fearful-me let possible outcomes play out in my mind and kept me from acting on my impulses.

I noticed an expression cross Mom's face, not sure what it meant.

Dad heard the one crutch hit the ground behind him and spun around. His eyes widened, and he jumped back away from me.

"What are you doing?"

"I'm stopping you from hurting Mom."

"You think she's better than me? I could tell you stories. She's no saint."

"I don't care what you have to say. You are not to hit her."

Dad must have sensed my fear because his eyes narrowed, and he edged toward me, spitting out his old threats. He focused on me like a wild animal preparing to pounce. Mom moved around and picked up the other crutch without Dad noticing. At the right moment, she told him to settle down or be settled down.

Dad looked back at her to see he now had two armed opponents with him in the middle. After more cursing and threats, Dad went into the house, pulled a bottle of beer from the refrigerator, sat in his chair in the living room, and lit a cigarette.

CHAPTER 5

THE TORMENT

Christmas 1964 was in sight, just a little more than a month away. This was going to be a special one. My brother, Kenny, married the neighbor girl, Phyllis, in August 1963 after returning home from the navy, and this past March they had a son. I had a new role for this holiday—uncle to a nine-month-old nephew. Now I had someone new to share my Christmas excitement with.

So many changes happened since last year's Christmas. Kenny, my hero and protector, came home from the navy. My relief at the possibilities of having him in the house to stand against Dad again turned too quickly into added torment. He returned more like Dad than the hero who left for basic training. Then he married and moved out of the house again. I watched as his new son sobered him. He cut back on his drinking and started taking his family to church. If Kenny could do that, surely Dad could. Could this be the Christmas God would grant my miracle?

A new family dynamic was rising from our ashes. Dad helped Phyllis learn the family game of Pinochle, complete with the customary teasing. And during the game, he often paused to play with baby Jeff. A warmth blanketed me as I watched him adjust to his new role as father-in-law and grandfather.

But just when my anticipation couldn't get any higher, Dad came home from work one night having drunk too many beers again. This time, he wasn't angry. He was worried. The place he had worked for as long as I could remember had announced it would close after Thanksgiving.

Panic gripped me. I tried to imagine Dad unemployed. *Will he spend his spare time at the bars?* Then I thought about Christmas and groaned. *Will we have any gifts under the tree? Will I get my binoculars*—the *one* present I had asked for? Being fourteen years old, I wanted real binoculars, not the toy ones I had in the past. Even the child's telescope I had never focused. I wanted to see up close the moon's craters, wild animals, and anything else I could capture in my lens. Now my hopes were fading.

In spite of the bleak future, Mom kept the family holiday traditions going. Thanksgiving lacked nothing in its usual feast. Afterwards, she made her usual Christmas candies. We went to her uncle's garage in Iuka to pick out a tree. Her best efforts almost made it look like our normal Christmas.

As I suspected, the holiday approached, but the tree sheltered fewer packages under its branches. Worse, I saw nothing that could be binoculars with my name on it.

I awoke early on Christmas day and slipped into the living room to check out the tree, just as I had as a child. I guess I was hoping Mom waited until I was asleep to put a surprise for me under it. Nothing had changed, so I went back to bed. When I heard Mom and Dad stirring, I got up again. Before Mom started breakfast, we sat in the living room and began opening presents.

After we opened our few presents, Dad got up from his chair. "There is one more." He disappeared into his bedroom. Returning, he handed me a small but heavy package with my name on it.

He never said a word as I sat dumbfounded. With Dad still unemployed, I had given up on getting anything more than the simple and inexpensive few presents I had already unwrapped. I was certain the binoculars were out of the question, but what else could be this size and this heavy?

"Aren't you going to open it?" Dad's lack of patience showed again.

I picked at the tape to carefully unwrap the box and save the paper.

"I just want you to know this is not a toy," he said. "You better take good care of it. I don't want to see you leaving it out to get broken or anything."

I couldn't believe I held 10x50 power binoculars in my hands. "Wow!" I said as I lifted them out of their leather carrying case. I hadn't asked nor expected anything close to this magnification. They had to have cost a lot, an amount that qualified as a sacrifice for Mom and Dad with the future so uncertain—a sacrifice I suddenly felt unworthy to receive.

A part of me wanted to tell him to return them and get his money back. "I will be very careful with them, Dad. Where did you find this power? The best I have seen in catalogs is 7x35 power."

"I kept telling the man in the store to show me something more until he said this was the best he had."

Somehow, Mom and Dad made it a good Christmas, after all.

That turned out to be the last Christmas in my boyhood home. The following March 1965, Dad and Mom sold our thirty acres and house for a little more than $8,000. For eight months, we rented a house in town across the street from Dad's brother Bob. Dad landed a job at a new factory that had moved into town. With a steady income restored, Dad fell back into his old routine of stopping at the bar after work and coming home drunk. Our family life started to resemble what it was before Dad lost his job. The surroundings were far different, but the daily routine too familiar. The only component missing was the hair-raising crossings over Crooked Creek bridge.

That fall, with their finances back on track, Dad and Mom bought a house on leased land in the oil fields. Again, we were about five miles out of town, but this time southwest instead of south of Salem.

The new neighborhood came complete with new friends who welcomed me into their circle. I found a place where I belonged. They had family dysfunctions and secrets, too. My new circle included two older brothers with motorcycles and their sister who was my age, and another high schooler who was on crutches because of cerebral palsy. He lived next door to us while the others were up the road less than a half-mile.

On my sixteenth birthday the following spring, I didn't realize Dad had been watching my new connections develop until he called out to me. "Get in the car."

He hadn't been drinking, so I figured it was safe to do as he said. "Where are we going, Dad?"

"To get you something for your birthday."

"Something?"

"You'll see."

Dad seemed to enjoy his little mystery. We didn't say much until he pulled into the local Honda dealer.

"I thought you would like to be able to ride with your friends."

"A motorcycle?"

He smiled.

My mind danced between elation and terror. *Do I want one? Well, yeah. This is awesome. But how comfortable will I be going fast on only two wheels? Hands controlling speed, clutch, lights, front brake, and turn signals while the feet control gears and rear brake. Reminds me of Grandma wanting to teach me piano—too many things to do with too many appendages at the same time. How hard is it to learn?*

"Dad, why? Can you afford it?"

"Don't worry about it. Just tell me which one you like."

It took me a while to believe this was happening. I just looked at him while I wrestled with my emotions. I appreciated what he was doing. I interpreted it to be his way of reaching out to me. But what I wanted, what I needed, was for him to stay sober, to say he loved me, to ask forgiveness for what he had done to us. I wanted to tell him so, but I had been conditioned against talking about anything personal with Dad, especially feelings.

I realized Dad's look had changed to impatience as I hadn't moved. He expected me to browse through the bikes and make a decision.

Each time he noticed me looking at a smaller bike, he nudged me toward a larger one so I would have enough speed for the highway and to keep up with my friends' larger bikes, but my fear of mastering it and the worry over the cost steered me toward the Honda 50—more of a scooter than a motorcycle. It had an automatic clutch, so I had one less function to synchronize. Its speed topped at forty-five with a good tailwind going downhill. Typical cruise speed held a comfortable thirty-five. Twenty-five cents filled the gas tank, and I could ride a hundred miles on that.

"This one," I said and watched his face fall. I think I disappointed Dad with my choice, but he probably decided it was better to buy something I would use.

I loved my scooter. That summer happened on it. Riding with my friends made for the best summer I ever remembered. It gave me new freedom. Every country road for miles around offered a new adventure to explore. The wind whisking my hair eroded my darkest thoughts, setting me free from the cares at home. This became my teen rebellion—a stay-at-home runaway. I ate and slept at home. Did my homework at home. Even played pinochle at home, but in every other way, I wasn't there when Dad was.

Each evening, after hours away from the house, I knew I would need to get back. The longer I was gone meant Mom had more time to face Dad alone. On my Honda, I could let the wind in my face swipe away the guilt pangs for abandoning her, but my ride had to end. Back home, as I reached for the doorknob, fear of what I might find on the other side sucker-punched me over and over.

Dad had landed another new job, another over-the-road trucking company. Like his previous ones, he often had longer runs that took him away from home for more than an overnight. He might get called to report for work at any time, day or night. Knowing he might have to haul an oil tanker behind him at highway speeds should have curtailed his drinking, but he let nothing stand between him and his bottles.

A few months into summer, Dad's spinster aunts decided to stop driving and gave me their car. In car years, it nearly qualified as an antique but with little more than fifty thousand miles on it. While their 1950 Plymouth wasn't cool like my classmates' cars, it kept me dry and warm in all kinds of weather and thus expanded my ability to go places.

When I wasn't hanging out with my neighborhood buddies, I spent time with my high school best friend, Chris, and his family. His mother, Dorothy, whom everyone called Dot, loved to tell about her life, and I loved listening to good stories. She told about what Chris and his brother, Chuck, were like as youngsters, and what it was like working in the army base mess hall when Chris's dad was there during the war, and how they lived in California and took trips up into the mountains. It was incredible to hear.

For some reason, she also shared about her alcoholic father, his terrible meanness, and the time he caused her little brother to drown. I found myself opening up my guarded secrets in response. I guess her sharing with me and making herself vulnerable made me believe I had found someone who would understand and not judge me. Being able to talk about it with someone released a great deal of my emotional pressure, and a kinship developed between us.

I also found a refuge. One Friday I had arrived at their house after dinner. Hours later, I knew I should have left and been home earlier, but Dad had returned that day from one of his trips. The old fear of what I might find when I got home invaded my mind. The later it got, the more fear tormented me with possibilities.

Dot interrupted my thoughts. "Why don't you spend the night, Huff?"

That scene happened several times, rarely when Dad was away, almost always when he was home. Later, I learned she invited me because I trembled when I said I should go home. I never noticed it, but she evidently saw something.

Without saying so, I adopted them as my rescue family. In them, I saw how a house with parents and teens should function and love one another—in real life, not some television comedy show. I never noticed any hesitance on their part with my intrusion. Instead, they made me feel as though I belonged—even by taking me on some family excursions. I am certain my high school years would have been different without the stability they introduced to me.

While they provided a much-needed escape, that momentary relief also planted a new terror in me. *What if Dad did something terrible to Mom while I was gone?* I felt tormented by the thought of returning home and finding Mom hurt—or worse. How would I live with myself knowing I chose to be gone when I could have prevented the worst had I been home? I felt guilty leaving Mom alone. At the same time, I was afraid my fear, anger, and bitterness might erupt into a lethal brew of unstoppable revenge. Walking away from my troubles seemed to be the best solution, but I couldn't help wondering if I could survive the crushing guilt if Dad killed Mom while I hid.

The terror gnawed at me. From month to month, I sensed its bites earlier and earlier. Instead of waiting until I reached for the door, my heart raced when I turned into our driveway, then before I turned down the road to our house, and even before I said goodbye to friends to start my ride home. Fear of being home kept me away until the fear of not going home became greater.

We had been in the oil-field house three years when the phone rang one night after Dad had staggered in and fallen asleep. With the phone in my hand, I called to him a few times and then nudged his shoulder. He sprang from the couch in a rage. Murder stared me down. His eyes flamed red. The lines on his forehead deepened. Of all the times I'd looked at his anger, hell and its demons never felt so close to me. "Dad! It's your boss on the phone."

He paused and squinted his eyes. He blinked a few times then jerked the phone out of my hand. Mom and I stood silent, exchanging nervous glances. Dad wrote notes of his boss's instructions then hung up. "I need up at four."

I looked at Mom and saw her tension leave. She nodded to say she would be sure to wake him on time.

With nothing more to say, he went to his bedroom and closed the door.

I went to my room, relieved I had escaped Dad's rage but complaining that God had not yet intervened in Dad's reign of terror. Where was God in all of this?

The two moves in 1965 interrupted our Sunday practice. Mom and I never found a church nearby where we felt at home. Truth be told, we tried only a couple of churches and then gave up. The God of power— the One who rolled back the waters of the Red Sea—didn't seem to be listening when I prayed. I didn't know if Mom was missing God or if she thought He could make a difference either, but I lost interest in Him and began looking for godlike power manifested elsewhere. The churches we were familiar with taught the mighty miracles of the Bible were necessary for the first century to establish the gospel. I believed in something more, so I searched for supernatural activity and found power in the occult. All the while, I continued to pray for Dad to stop drinking. I prayed in case God was listening. So desperate to have Dad's reign of terror over us end, I told God to strike him down physically if necessary—anything to get him to stop drinking.

But something had to give. And it had to give soon.

I just didn't know it would be something within me.

CHAPTER 6

WINDS OF CHANGE

On the surface, my high school years produced good things. I had my last foot surgery before entering my freshman year so I no longer had to miss school to go to the clinic. A band trip at the end of my junior year took me to the Bahamas. And I had a monologue in my senior year band variety show that won me an extra curtain call. The transportation I was gifted—the Honda and the 1950 Plymouth—allowed me to get a job as a stockboy at a local department store, which I thoroughly enjoyed. Summers were filled with exploring every country lane I encountered and hanging out with friends. But one excursion took me to a place I never wanted to be and nearly ruined a friendship.

One of my friends, Julie, and I were both excellent students and competed against each other in band. She sat first chair trumpet to my second chair. She and her sister also had gotten a small motorcycle and joined with me on riding the roads and trails. On one of our trips, she insisted on introducing me to a special friend of hers. Her excitement built my expectations.

She led me down several roads and turns, ending on a lane toward a Lake Centralia shoreline. Partway down the lane, we stopped to talk to a scruffy man about my dad's age who motored around in a large electric wheelchair, the type Raymond Burr rode in his role in the television series *Ironside*. This was her special friend she wanted me to meet. In the brief conversation we had, I observed him to be just like my dad, maybe even worse. Besides being a drinker, he said things that ranged between inappropriate for mixed company to outright lewd. He had a friendly, disarming smile, but no overtures toward me could overcome the image of Dad's worst moments.

I told my friend I never wanted to go back and visit the man again. We cut our ride short that day, and all the way home, I wrestled with questions and possible answers. How could she be so gullible to fall for his flirtation? Did she like it? That's not the girl I thought she was. He openly talked of drunken parties. How could she be attracted to that? I couldn't imagine why she would admire him so.

Maybe she isn't the girl I thought she was. What dark secrets has she hidden from me?

We met up for a few more rides that summer. Nothing more was ever mentioned about her friend. I tried to focus on what was happening in the moment, leaving the questions behind us in the clouds of dust kicked up by our scooters. School started in the fall and took us separate ways.

About a year later, a family moved a trailer into an empty lot across from our house. The father introduced me to the world of CB radios and helped me get one of my own. I got my license, call letters, a CB handle, and a host of new unseen friends. A few became favorites, including a feisty, funny character who called himself the Mayor of Lake Centralia. I heard about monthly meetings in the area of local CBers that I couldn't wait to attend. I wanted so much to put faces to the voices of my newest crop of friends.

I got to the meeting early so I could meet as many as I could when they arrived. I recognized Jolly the moment he spoke. I figured out who Cotton was. He had chosen his handle in reference to his thick white head of hair. When Tac (short for tachometer) walked in, I was shocked to see he had been my seventh-grade teacher. But where was the Mayor?

He never showed. Another month of chitchat and exchanging wisecracks deepened my desire to meet the man who held such respect among the CBers and who had a quick wit I enjoyed sparring with.

When the time for the next meeting came around, he told me he would surely be there.

Again I arrived early and started greeting different ones, while all the time watching and listening for the Mayor. Then I heard his voice behind me. We had planned to meet and sit at the same table to get to know each other better. I turned to see him, and my breath caught in my throat. There sat the man and his wheelchair whom I determined never to see again. How could we have become such friends? His radio persona stood in sharp contrast to the man I had met on the road.

"I have a table for us over here," Jolly called out, making me feel trapped. I forced the memories of our times on the radio together joking and teasing each other and others over the airwaves to overshadow the memory of my first meeting with him. Everyone found their seats and settled in for the meeting while the usual radio banters interrupted serious business.

I learned that evening the official name of The Mayor of Lake Centralia: Charlie Strain. Jolly served as an intermittent caregiver for Charlie helping him to bed or getting him up and around first thing in the morning. At the meeting, Charlie was the same man as the voice on the radio. The bantering around the table that night weakened my resolve and resistance. The wall I had built against him could no longer stand. By the end of the meeting, Charlie secured a promise from me to visit him at his home.

The memory of my first meeting Charlie boiled up as I neared his house. How had I let him talk me into this? I knew I had to make him understand my terms of friendship. *Right. How am I going to do that?*

I hesitantly knocked, and the radio voice filtered through the door. "Come in, the door isn't locked."

The first thing I saw when I opened the door was Charlie's smile. Something about it made it beguiling and disarming, but at the same time welcoming. Big as it was, it spread across his face like the wings of an eagle stretching out to catch the updraft and soar.

"Sherlock! You made it." Charlie always called me by my CB handle since we were both named Charles.

The three-room house was built especially for his large, electric wheelchair. The open floor plan had lower cabinets and counters. Furniture kept at a minimum, but comfortable. Looking around, I could tell we were alone. This was my opportunity to share with him about my dad and how drinking upset me.

Charlie's countenance softened to communicate compassion and total honesty. "Thank you for sharing. I understand. I will make you this promise. I will never ask you to fetch me a beer from the refrigerator, and I will never drink in excess when you are around." He also promised to tell me ahead of time if he thought he wanted to get drunk so I could stay away.

The first visit turned into a second, then a third, and eventually into being his permanent caregiver until I left for college. He taught me how to work with his manual lift to get him out of bed, onto the toilet, dressed, and into his chair. From that point, he could take care of himself until bedtime.

I spent the days learning to play dominoes and listening to his stories.

"I grew up in Kansas during the Great Depression. When I could, I would stop at the pool hall and gamble on games, either shooting pool or playing dominoes for money. I got so good that the owner asked if I wanted to play for the house. I made some good money those days there and at the golf course where I caddied."

He still played dominoes as if money were on the table. Except he taught strategy while he played. I knew I had mastered the game when I bested him. He cussed that I had been lucky in the draw and any other excuses for why I won, then laughed and congratulated me on a good game.

Over time, I learned that he often had that same response to other situations. He could explode with hot, withering anger at someone messing up in some way. At first, we were ready to jump out of his way in case he tried to run over us with his chair. Then he would give his gut-busting laughter and point out some humor we all missed. That was probably a left-over from his boxing days.

"Twice I won the title of light-weight boxing champion in Kansas. I once got into a fight with a man almost double my size. I used my technique on him. I squared off against him then when I saw the opportunity, I slapped his face. This surprised him because I didn't punch him. He thought I wasn't being serious or that I was making fun of him. After a few more slaps, he became angry at my openhanded insults and lost his concentration. I knew at that point the win was mine." Charlie controlled his temper while making use of an opponent's lack of control.

"I was a year away from pro golf when I noticed something wrong with my swing, so I went to a doctor to be checked out. After running a battery of tests, he told me I had muscular dystrophy, a slow advancing kind. My golfing career was over before it got started. The army would not take me because of the disability. So I packed up and moved here to southern Illinois and got a job in the oil field."

Charlie kept working that job until he had to walk with two canes and climb the tank ladders using only his arms because his legs would not hold his weight. The company at that point forced him to retire. He saw that as an opportunity to learn a new trade and sent off for a correspondence course for watch repair. One of his friends built an oak desk in the corner of his bedroom, designed for access with his wheelchair, and he earned extra cash fixing watches. He couldn't be inactive.

"There are two times, only two, when I feel bad about this muscular dystrophy. I hate it when I can't stand for the national anthem or when a woman enters the room."

Charlie kept his promises to me. More than just appeasing me, he respected me for my convictions and for sticking to them. Most of my exchanges with older adults left me feeling like they saw me as a kid still lacking in life experiences, or as the old saying puts it, "Still wet behind the ears." Charlie made me feel like his equal. My self-esteem grew that summer.

Charlie brought up the subject of my dad sometime around the middle of that summer. He shared examples of men who came home from the war seriously changed and said I should consider the possibilities with my dad. He dropped the subject then and never brought it up again.

I considered how my attitude toward Charlie had totally reversed from our first meeting. The thought of something like that happening between Dad and me seemed impossible. Maybe I could be a little more understanding, but unless Dad became more like Charlie and saw me as an equal, nothing would ever change between us. But for the moment, I relaxed, being thankful for another refuge away from my house.

Once again staying true to his promise, one weekend, Charlie told me I could spend the time at home. He had other friends who would take care of him, and they would probably be drinking.

"When do I need to make myself scarce? Do you need me to help you tonight, or is someone coming today?"

"I can get someone for tonight. You've been here several days in a row. You should probably check in with your mom and dad."

When I got home, Mom asked how my time with Charlie had been, how he was doing, and anything else she could think of for conversation. I loved that we had such a relationship, but overall, nothing had changed in our home environment. Mom still busied herself with keeping the house. Dad still came home in a foul mood and drunk. I still tried to keep distance between us.

The next morning, however, Mom rushed Dad to the hospital. He woke up spitting up blood and with slurred speech.

After running tests, the doctor sat down with Dad. "Do you drink alcohol?"

"A few beers at night."

"You have to stop. The beer has eroded the lining of your stomach. You are very lucky that only a small vessel burst rather than several or a larger one. You could have bled out. Other tests show you also had a mild stroke. If you want to live longer, you must stop drinking."

Dad cut back on his drinking habit. Though he couldn't completely stop, I thanked God for even that much. But it didn't last. After a few weeks with no health crisis, Dad returned to his old ways.

About that time, when I was home from Charlie's again, Dad got up for breakfast and sat at the table. He seemed unusually quiet, then something happened. He looked different. Mom asked if he was okay, but he couldn't answer. He had difficulty saying anything. The right side of his face sagged. This signaled a severe stroke. Mom called for an ambulance.

At the hospital, the doctor ordered a pint of blood be taken. It came out thick like molasses. The doctor told us the alcohol had affected his spleen, making his blood so thick.

The doctor put Dad on blood-thinner medication while ordering a pint of blood drawn from him every other week at first, then monthly until his blood cell count normalized. Each month the count improved, but it took six months for the cell count to be normal and stable. The heavy-drinker body odor that oozed from Dad's pores diminished in parallel grades until it was gone at six months, too.

After the local hospital had done all they could for him, they sent him to the veterans' hospital in Marion, Illinois—an hour from our house—for physical therapy. He had lost use of his right hand, right leg, and much of his speech. After intense therapy, he regained enough strength to stand on his right leg, but he walked by stepping with his left foot and dragging his right. He had trouble putting words together and sometimes used the wrong word. He usually swore when that happened and either tried again or shut up in anger.

I had said to the Lord to do whatever was necessary to get Dad to stop drinking. Was this the answer to my prayer? Had I moved God's hand to this? If so, only part of my prayers had been answered. Dad no longer drank. However, his heart never changed. He never desired to go to church. In fact, the stroke locked him in his drunken mentality. He continued to exhibit his monster traits, only now while sober. His physical impairment added to his frustration and short temper. Fear still resided with us, only not as severe. Dad had mellowed a little toward us. Without any thanks or anything said to suggest he appreciated our help, he relaxed and accepted our attempts to help him.

Kenny did little to help us. He worked full time, and his family had grown to include two more boys, the youngest being a newborn. What extra time he had, he spent hunting or fishing.

Mom continued doing what she had always done—serve him. I, on the other hand, faced my own adjustments. All my life, my approach to Dad had formed into two strategies: keep a good distance between us and cry out to God for anything to make him stop drinking.

Condemning whispers of guilt blended with my pity for Dad's condition to create an unholy compassion, which I let cover my anger and fear like a scab. Outwardly, I helped Mom tend to Dad's needs. Inwardly, I wrestled with my anger and guilt. Dad didn't change. I still saw the monster within him even without the beer. And to make matters worse, now I had to serve him.

I argued point and counterpoint in my mind over what my response should be through this new family dynamic. *He did this to himself. Mom and others tried to get him to stop, to seek out help. Now he's reaping what he sowed. He's at our mercy. I want payback . . . but . . . he's my dad.* I had always wanted his approval and love. I remembered Charlie's words about men coming back from the war. Could this be an opportunity for reconciliation? To receive that approval and love—that respect—from Dad? What, if anything, had changed?

I couldn't find my way out of my divided soul toward Dad. I hated him but wanted to love him at the same time. I saw my struggle in perfect clarity one day as winter settled in. I woke early on a Saturday morning—much earlier than desired—to a loud drumming. My mind first tried to recognize the sound and to figure out its source. Thoughts wormed through my confusion on what to say to the neighbor waking us up in such a manner.

Lying there sorting my thoughts, I became aware of my heart's rapid, strong beat. I reached up and felt the veins in my neck. They stood out like stiff straws under my skin. The banging drum was my heart. Each pump forcing my blood and swelling my veins and arteries created a booming in my ears.

Dad, Mom, and I had been having headaches for a few days, but neither of us ever had a fever. It couldn't be the flu as we suspected, but what else could it be?

Carbon monoxide.

I don't know where that thought came from, but it came as clear to my mind as if spoken. I could think of only one simple way to test it: get outside for some fresh air. I stood up and slipped on my robe. The room wobbled and spun. Dropping back on my bed, I waited for the room to stand still. The thought went through my mind that if it was carbon monoxide, I couldn't wait.

I reached out for furniture, doors, and walls—anything that could help me move toward the back door. Nearly through the kitchen, the room spun out of control again, and my legs turned to rubber. I collapsed over the sink. Only a few feet remained between me and clean air. Holding firmly to the counter, I tried to stand. Not yet. I collapsed with my full weight again over the sink. A few moments passed. One more attempt got me to the door and outside. The brisk November air stung my lungs.

Clutching the porch post to keep from falling, I felt strength flow into my legs. The drumming stopped. The veins in my neck returned to normal. I bent over to touch my toes. Dizziness was gone. It took only a minute or two for full recovery. The evidence convinced me the voice in my head was right.

I propped the door open to let out the bad air in the house. After taking a deep breath, I went back into the house and shut the furnace off. Fear of what I might find on the other side of Mom and Dad's bedroom door gripped me and stopped me before knocking. *Why have they not gotten up already? They are usually up before me. Could Dad's heart survive the extra stress?*

I tapped on the door. "Mom?" *That came out weaker and shakier than I intended.*

No answer. I knocked again with a little more urgency in my voice. "Mom."

"Yes."

She's alive. "Is Dad okay?"

"Yes. Why?"

"We may have carbon monoxide in the house, so I turned the furnace off."

A repairman later confirmed we had a large rust hole in our heat exchanger that allowed the poisonous gas to escape into our living space instead of safely venting out the chimney. We had no basement, so our furnace was suspended from the floor joists in the middle of our four-room house. He guessed the strong westerly winds in the night pushed the gas under my bedroom where it seeped through the floorboards and into my room. That gave a plausible explanation why the gas affected me while Mom and Dad had no ill effects. I was just grateful my guardian angel wasn't away on vacation that night.

For several days, the events of that day played out in my mind in a constant loop. The fear that stood in my way outside the bedroom door was vaguely familiar but so different from what I had been living with. Instead of fearing Mom would be lying dead from some heinous act, I feared both might be dead from a tragic accident. When had been the last time I feared for Dad's safety? More than nine years before when he raced toward the wrecked car covered in a thick cloud.

From that moment, I looked at Dad differently. Serving him became less out of duty and more out of compassion. However, I still saw the monster lying low, waiting, always looking for an issue to force his authority over us. Even though Charlie, the Mayor, had sparked a renewed hope in me, I couldn't shake the love-hate battle in my heart and mind.

Years of anger for what he had done, bitterness for his blindness to our pain, and hatred for his abusive control of us stifled what little compassion I had for him. I knew it would take a miracle to change all that. Unfortunately, I had concluded God was no longer in the miracle business—at least not for us.

CHAPTER 7

LOST

Summer 1970 ushered in more upheavals. In June, I graduated from our community college with top honors in an associate in arts degree. I successfully enrolled for the fall semester at the University of Illinois, Champaign-Urbana. Envisioning a homeboy-makes-good-despite-rough-start story, I planned on two more years of college and then graduate school. I wanted to make Mom proud. I wanted my second parents, Lee and Dorothy (Dot) proud. And, honestly, showing up those who slighted me down through the years also claimed a part of my imagination.

Eleven months had passed since Dad's stroke. He had no use of his right arm, walked by dragging his right leg, and his speech was still broken with pauses and wrong words. We gave up all hope that he was ever going to get any better. That left Mom needing to become the decision maker. Her first major decision severed us from the family farm and our family history. She could not manage our house and the farmhouse Dad bought from his aunts. With her dream of adding on to the farmhouse and moving there crashed, she put it up for sale. A few weeks later, she also sold the house we were living in.

We moved back into Salem.

Mom reasoned that Dad's medical condition required us to be closer to doctors and the hospital, and I agreed. Living in town also ended Dad's control over her. Mom often complained that we lived in the country because of Dad. She believed he wanted to keep her at home taking care of the house, tending the garden, and fixing his dinners—whether he ever made it home to eat them or not. Most of the time we had only one car, so when Dad drove himself to work—which was most often—Mom had no way to go anywhere. Captive in her home. A simple matter of control over her. That era was now history.

The move into town was only about a five-mile shift. It should not have impacted me, but it drew my attention to the other changes the year brought to me, family, and friends, magnifying in my mind the aftermath. My neighbors who had filled my days were no longer a walk next door. My high school buddies and I rarely got together. If they were not away at different colleges, they were married and had full-time jobs to occupy their time. My cousins, quite naturally, were caught in the same demanding activities so fewer came each year to the family reunions. All this set in a new round of separation and isolation for me. I had to find a new circle of friends to help me through.

I tried to focus on the good things happening. My school plans were working out. Dad no longer drank. Fear of what he might do lessened. A coexistence worked into our lives. The house was okay. It was neat and clean, though it was the smallest one I had ever lived in.

Hoping to find something to keep redirecting my thoughts, I checked for any of my friends on the CB radio. All I could hear was noise, no local chatter. I gave up on that and tried settling in on watching television. But summer afternoons had little to offer—soap operas, game shows, or old movies.

Leaving the channel on a game show I really didn't care about put some background noise in the room. My thoughts drifted to wondering if, now that my dad's situation had changed, a father/son bond had a chance of developing.

Raised voices in the kitchen interrupted my daydream.

"I have an appointment to get my hair done," Mom said.

"I don't care. I said you are not leaving this house."

I turned to see what was happening right when Dad hit Mom. I sprang from the couch and reached the kitchen as Dad was coming out. Without hesitation, I slapped him across the face! His glasses sailed across the room. Stunned by my action, I stood silent but for my heavy breathing, unsure what to do next.

Dad staggered backward, then glared at me. For the first time, though, I saw human anger instead of the demonic I had witnessed for years. "I'm your dad."

"Yes, and she's my mom. I told you before to never hit her."

"Get out. My. House."

I remembered the letter my sister-in-law, Phyllis, told me about. In it, Dad had crushed Kenny's dream of college and teaching math. And Kenny had returned from the navy like Dad in his drinking.

"I heard you kicked Kenny out of the house. You were his reason for joining the navy early. He rolled over too easy. I'm not leaving. You will continue to take care of my needs until I graduate or maybe longer if Mom needs me."

He grabbed me and started pushing me toward the front door. The strength he still had surprised me, though his stricken right side gave me a distinct advantage. After I pushed him back and planted him on the couch, he glared and tried to reclaim his alpha-dog position. "Better watch it."

"Don't hit Mom and we should be okay." Even saying the words, I wondered, *Will it? Or will Dad just wait until I'm not around to get violent with her?* Then my future plans came into question. *Should I be heading to the university, leaving her alone with him?*

The rest of the summer passed without further conflict. Dad even went with me to haul my things to my dorm room. We didn't talk much during the three-hour drive, but I sensed he enjoyed being back on the road again.

At the school, I found my room and moved my minimal college survival supplies in. My roommate hadn't arrived yet. All I knew of him was that he was fresh from the navy. Perhaps we could have some common ground since Kenny had been a sailor too. The thought gave me a thread of hope for a good year.

As soon as I met him, it became clear he was ready to let loose after his military service. Studying was not high on his radar. He connected with others on the floor who focused on partying. Each night, he stumbled back to our room smelling of stale beer and cigarettes.

The smell and his attitudes raised images of my life with Dad before his stroke. My tremors started again. Unlike in my high school years, I noticed them. Releasing my pent-up anger on him crossed my mind at least once. Familial ties didn't stand in my way, but I couldn't. When I thought I had tolerated the worst, he started creating his own hard cider in the room. The smell of a brewery lay heavy in the room and layered with the stale beer stench he wore when he came in.

Being trapped in the tight confines of our dorm room with all I hated triggered old nightmares. I lost all focus. My grades plummeted. When I asked the floor resident advisor for a new room assignment, he told me nothing was available. Maybe next semester.

I should have gone home and tried again in the summer or the next fall. But my stubbornness locked me in place. Perhaps the following semester would usher in a new roommate and change everything for me. But I needed immediate help and had no friends to lean on.

I wished I were back sitting across from Charlie at his table. He had done so much to boost my confidence. I knew he would have some bit of wisdom to share that would get me focused again. He had that way about him. But a letter from Mom informed me that Charlie had died. A large piece of my safety net was now gone.

The second semester started off with a positive change. I got a new roommate, Jim, on an entirely different floor. Though he and I hit it off great, that first semester in hell had left me badly shaken. I couldn't pull myself back together. By the end of the year, after the university issued final grades, they sent me a letter informing me I could continue next year but on probationary status. Having always been in the top 10 percent of my class through fourteen years of schooling, I crumbled. I didn't know how to pull out of my tailspin.

I visited Dorothy and Lee, my best friend's parents, once that summer after my first year at the university, hoping to recapture some portion of support and safety. I felt too ashamed to let them know my latest trauma. Dorothy gave me a wallet-sized photo of a family portrait they had taken earlier. She had insisted they have it done because they might never have another chance. Their tight-knit family was being pulled apart. Chris had left for the navy, and Chuck had started college away from home. While I enjoyed my visit, I returned home in no better mindset.

I tried recreating myself. My newest friends introduced me to mixed drinks. The drinks didn't smell like beer, and I discovered I liked their taste. I let my hair grow out and changed my wardrobe to something trendier. The following semester, returning to the same dorm, a guy from my floor called out, "Hey, there's good ol' Charley Huff. Wait. That's a new Charley Huff. What happened to you?"

The fall semester of my senior year started with a renewed zeal to prove what I could do. Jim and I were roommates again. I loved my classes. However, my euphoria imploded midway through the first semester. In late October, I contracted mononucleosis and missed more than a week of classes. Then I received a letter from my girlfriend of two years calling everything off. When I went home that weekend, Mom told me Dad had filed for divorce. But the next weekend broke the final band holding me together. Dorothy and Lee were killed in a car crash. My safety net now lay in shreds.

I went home for the funeral and ended up staying that night at the house with Chris and Chuck. I don't know who needed support the most. While we were together, we put on a good show at moving forward.

On Sunday I headed back to school. Chris expressed he was leaving as soon as possible to report back on base. Chuck seemed determined to return to his classes as well.

The sun rose Monday morning, but my heart still lay flatlined in misery. I called home. Mom said Chuck pulled out of school to handle all the estate details and the home. His nineteenth birthday was less than two weeks away. I couldn't let him have it totally alone.

As for my own classes, my mind was once again mush. I couldn't focus on anything but my circumstances and Chuck's. I left my dorm room to speak with the dean of liberal arts studies. He sat behind his desk with his arms resting on it. As I unrolled the month's events, I noticed he leaned backward more with each thing I told.

When I got to the crash, he rocked forward, causing his chair to bang. "My goodness, is there anything else? Here's the thing. You are past the time to pull out without an incomplete/failure put on your record, but I'm waiving that. It will be like you weren't here. Go home. Do what you must."

With that, my college career, plans, and dreams ended.

A significant part of my heart turned cold toward God. What good was it to keep me from dying from the many trips home from town with my drunken father driving? Why save me from the shotgun incident, the carbon monoxide poisoning, and so many other times? Why—if I wasn't going to be allowed to make something of myself?

I had already put God into a ratty box in the attic of my heart. Losing Dot and Lee ripped me apart. I justified my anger against God. Yet something within me believed my best friend's parents were with Jesus in glory. Doubts and anger toward God for letting these things happen kept me from having the peace I wanted.

One thought in the mess brought me some relief. Dad had removed himself from our lives. I didn't have to worry about Mom's safety anymore. And except for occasional family gatherings, I didn't have to spend time with him. I didn't have to check in on him. I had time to coast.

Chris did return to the navy after the funeral, and instead of having a court-appointed guardianship, Chuck had to be declared an adult by the court to handle the estate. I moved in with him for mutual support in grief.

We both found jobs in the area and, in time, began to crawl out of our slump. We struck up new friendships and started doing some double dating. After a few months, I realized I hated my job as an assistant credit manager in a furniture store. The classy title for a debt collector did nothing for easing my conscience about having to be the bad guy. I tried my best, but after a few months of beating myself up over it, I hit upon a plan.

That summer of 1972, I asked for time off, contacted my good college roommate Jim, and asked if I could visit him and his family for a week. Their farm was not far from Quincy, Illinois, across the Mississippi from Hannibal, Missouri. They welcomed me almost to the point of embarrassing me. Jim planned my whole vacation, including a trip to see Mark Twain's home and Tom Sawyer's cave in Hannibal. One thing he hadn't considered were his father's plans for the days I was there. Certain farm chores had to be done without delay. Guests had to fit around the farm's needs.

When his dad got us up early the first morning to help him castrate pigs, Jim was mortified. "Dad, Charley came for a vacation."

I wasn't going to be the reason for a rift between the two of them. Besides, I came to find out what I was going to do with my job. Experiencing the hard farm work was good therapy for me. "Jim, please, I came for a change. I need new experiences. It's fine with me. Let's do this."

The other event none of us planned on was the tornado that grazed us, knocking down half a tree the day before I was to leave. It fell across the road, so as soon as the storm passed, we were out cutting and pulling the tree off the road. Jim felt horrible about how my vacation went.

Almost with tears of gratitude, I told him the time had been perfect. I hadn't felt this good in months. The hard work while helping my host family held rewards that sightseeing would never come close to. Discovering joy in working opened my mind to see what I had to do. As soon as I returned home, I gave my employer my notice, not knowing where my next job would take me.

Because my work history involved some aspect of retail, I scoured the want ads for any related opportunity. One of the first interviews I went on landed me a job as a sale's clerk in a men's clothing store in Marion, Illinois, in the lower tip of the state. Gleaning some necessary things my mom said I could have (dishes, silverware, towels, minimal furniture) and packing my things from Chris and Chuck's house, I moved into an apartment by myself.

Knowing Chuck's attitude toward anything supernatural, I had laid my dabbling aside while we lived together. Being alone, I needed something to fill my off-work time. Without a CB radio set up, I turned to occult activities, which I'd played around with briefly in college. In my searches, I came across a study program that promised to increase a person's sixth sense ability. Occasionally, I had experiences that indicated the system was working, such as the time I received a letter from Jim.

Jim and I maintained contact through writing each other. I especially enjoyed his letters since he always wrote entertaining news. As soon as I touched the envelope I received one particular day, I sensed a heavy foreboding come over me. I had no reason to expect anything since only a couple of months had passed from my vacation with them. Everyone was fine when I left. Something told me his letter contained bad news. My thoughts went first to Jim's dad. Jim's mom and dad had children later in life. He was a big man so his having a heart attack would not have surprised me. But then I sensed the letter held news about his mother. Sure enough, doctors found an aneurysm in his mother's brain that needed emergency surgery.

Though the surgery went well, a couple days later an X-ray showed that the clip to seal off the aneurysm had slipped. The doctors had to repeat the surgery. It too finished without any difficulty and was deemed successful. However, the stress of both surgeries and anesthesia proved too much for her body. She slipped away into eternity.

The pain and grief I shared with him were offset by the satisfaction of the spiritual sensitivity that forewarned me about the letter contents.

Pride over having a power resident in me above anything I had seen in churches soared and pushed me to pursue the occult even more.

At the clothing store, I laughed inwardly about the customers I kept getting who tried to save my poor lost soul. Oddly enough, they all seemed to be Baptists. With the crises behind and a new future before me, I didn't think I needed any saving, and I certainly was not eager to become anyone's coup. So I devised a tactic to scare them all away from making me another victory notch for them. At the end of the sales transaction, I'd say, "It's been great getting to know you. I think you will be happy with your selection. Remember, if you have any problems, come back and see me."

"Sure thing, and thank you. You were very helpful," they'd reply. "If you are not doing anything this Sunday, how about coming with me to our church service?"

"Thanks. Maybe I will. And if you ever want to hang out, go for a coke or something, stop by my apartment. I'll write down my address for you."

Though they offered a look of surprise, they'd say, "Maybe I will. Thanks."

I was certain they were about as sincere as I was. Either way, I could ferret out those who really took an interest in me as opposed to those who just wanted to make a show of their outreach successes. I wondered if they pictured my bachelor place as the proverbial den of iniquity.

My defensive scheme worked beautifully until one evening when someone knocked on my door. My young customer from the day before stood waiting to be invited in. He had called my bluff. Being close in age gave us some camaraderie that helped us pick up our discussions where we left off at the store. We talked maybe an hour or more, and not about weather or sports. He got to know me—what foods I liked and my music preferences, what television shows I enjoyed, what I did for entertainment, and where I was from. He shared much the same things about himself, and we surprised each other with how well suited we were for becoming friends.

Toward the end of the evening, he admitted that his friends and family called him Spanky. Then he cleared his throat and said he needed to go, but before leaving, he reminded me of my promise. I agreed, and Sunday morning, I sat beside him in his small Baptist church in the next community north of Marion.

His church service followed the pattern of what I remembered from church services in my youth, and the content had changed little in my absence. I did, however, notice sincerity in their words that I had not been around in years. They weren't collecting coup; their interest in me was real. From that moment on, God began bringing Scripture verses to mind from my boyhood years. I wrestled with the passages because they didn't fit into the philosophy I had developed—a mixture of the occult with the Scripture. *Those verses can't mean what it sounds like.* I had twisted words and meanings until the blood, the sacrifice, and even the resurrection had been washed out of them. I believed those things were symbolic of love and nothing more.

Spanky never backed down. He did the unimaginable by visiting me again. Naturally, I felt obligated to attend his church again. Having a friendship develop met a deep need I had so I relaxed my defenses to see where this path might take me.

After befriending Spanky, I met my next-door neighbor. He attended a church in Marion, almost walking distance from my apartment. Another Baptist, of course. He told me about their youth group meetings they called "Drop-In" on Tuesday evenings and invited me to attend. He told me he had a girl in mind I should meet. Intrigued by both the meeting *and* the girl, I went with him, but she wasn't there that night.

Jesus continued to challenge me, as if pressing me into a corner, with the verses quoted in the sermons. One by one, I deflected them with my occult understanding. They increasingly became more difficult until God reminded me of one more verse: "I am the way, the truth, and the life. No one comes to the Father except through Me" (John 14:6, NKJV). Jesus unequivocally saying He was the only way stumped me. I could find no way of understanding that verse except as it was. I faced three ways to respond. One: that it held a hidden meaning, which I hadn't yet figured out. Two: that Jesus was a superb conman and liar. Or three: that Jesus' statement about Himself was the truth—meaning that all my occult wisdom was rubbish and I was the greatest fool in all creation for having followed it. I went to bed tormented by that verse, until Jesus woke me up with a vision of me falling.

I sat up feeling terrified. Relieved it was only a dream, I lay back and closed my eyes. As soon as I did, the room started falling again. I opened my eyes, and it stopped. Each time I closed them, I was free-falling again. Because of my occult activity, I was familiar with visions and concluded I was *experiencing* a vision instead of observing one. I decided to close my eyes, let the fall happen, and pay attention to all my senses.

I realized I wasn't falling through open sky. Instead, I was in an enclosure. I was sure I would feel the walls if I reached out for them. It seemed round like a silo or a well, but bottomless. I looked up and saw a man in a white robe at the top. Somehow I knew it was Jesus.

"Depart from me you worker of iniquity," He said to me. "I never knew you."

I rolled over and fell for real—right onto the floor. I was just told the third possible understanding of that one verse was the truth, meaning how big a fool I had been.

While I had gone forward at a revival meeting when I was nine and was baptized, I did so believing what I was told. I was a sinner because the Bible said all have sinned. I believed Jesus died on the cross for those sins of mine and rose again that I might also live. But I never felt the weight of sin. I never fully understood how it was a part of me. Not until I was shown the gravity of mocking Jesus and the Word did I really repent. The following Tuesday, I went to Drop-In a changed man. It was time to see what Jesus could do with my life.

CHAPTER 8

NEW PATH AND OLD RUT

On my second visit to Drop-In in February 1973, I had two desires drawing me there. I was now caught up in experiencing Jesus in a new way, and I was curious about the girl my neighbor was so adamant I meet. My neighbor Jim, not to be confused with my old college roommate Jim, explained Cindy missed the previous week because her parents moved to Aurora, a town in the upper part of the state near Chicago, after making arrangements for her to stay in Marion to graduate with her friends. They found a suitable and agreeable family in town whom she could live with to finish her final three months of her senior year.

Moments after walking into Drop-In, Jim dragged me across the room to introduce me to that girl. I started a conversation cordially but friendly. The five-to-six years that separated us formed a void before me for talking topics. In my stumbling attempt, Cindy kept me from being dead on arrival as she easily moved from one topic to the next. My awkwardness lost its grip on me and slipped to the floor.

My first impression of her was how her sweet, simple beauty gave way to her enthusiasm and openness to making new friends. We spoke briefly, but with the meeting starting, Cindy and I purposed to reconnect afterwards to talk. I could hardly wait for the meeting to be over.

Our later conversation flowed with unbelievable ease. In a few minutes, we discovered we had several common interests, like live theater, old comedies, and definitely movies over sports. She made our encounter fun. More than any other thing about her, I loved her laughter. By that I mean her gut-busting laughter. In those moments, she pursed her lips to stifle the gaffaw that wanted to come out. Trapped inside, it seemed to ricochet around in her body, escaping occasionally in little shrieks. I tried everything I could to make her laugh that way again and again. The greatest thing I noticed about her was how much she relaxed me. I didn't have to pretend to be someone I wasn't. And for the next few days, I found I couldn't get her out of my mind.

I struggled against those thoughts. She was, after all, only seventeen to my twenty-three years. Jesus had just turned my life around, and I had no idea where it was now going. About two years before, I experienced what I said I never wanted—a sweetheart breakup. When I was in high school, I had watched friends go through relationships and painful breakups. I determined never to let that happen. Even though I had stopped going to church for so many years, I had still prayed about things that mattered to me. And many times I'd asked God to keep me from those experiences by revealing to me who I was going to marry when I met the person. I thought I had found it with my first girlfriend, but it wasn't to be. And now this young girl has turned my heart. I couldn't deny how she made me feel.

Only a couple weeks had passed when I decided to ask her for a date. The old me would never have been a good match for any chance of a relationship with her, but we met after Jesus recreated me. I had to see if being with only her and not the whole Drop-In crowd made a difference in our conversations and connection.

I was still struggling financially so I had struck upon the idea of a picnic and exploring the national forest preserve in the area. After Cindy agreed to go on a date with me, I remembered that prayer and the image of a girl in a dream who seemed like an answer to that prayer. Slender, oh so cute, and fun.

Spring had come a little early that year in southern Illinois so I scheduled our date a few days out for one of my days off, hoping it would be dry and warm. In the days leading up to our March 5 date, I noticed things happening that I believed only God could orchestrate. We would not have met had her parents insisted she move with them to Aurora. That is unless I had yielded to the unending advice to go to Aurora to seek work for better pay. Would God have made a way for us to meet there? That possibility kept sweeping through my mind.

A week before our date, my neighbor Jim went with me for a walk. During our time together, I began unloading on him my internal struggle. I told him about my high school prayer and dream, about the attributes I had listed for a perfect mate that Cindy fulfilled (except for playing piano), and other remarkable circumstances. A part of me was excited about the possibilities while the rest of me wallowed in the fear of another buildup and breakup. Jim suggested maybe God would give direction with a fleece as He done for Gideon in the Bible. He and I then became encased in a flower scent like the sachet Cindy wore. But at the end of February, no flowers were out of the ground yet. That too felt like a sign to me.

With all these "signs," I became convinced Jesus was honoring that forgotten prayer. I believed so strongly that I panicked and nearly skipped the date without calling her or giving her a reason. But I knew that would be rude, so I went, but I was miserable trying to act natural, while knowing it was all an act—and probably a very bad one. Two hours the torture lasted until our date finally drew to a close. I didn't know what to do with the thought that God was saying she could be my wife one day. Afraid that I had ruined our date by trying too hard to be the same as at the Drop-In meetings, I didn't know if I should try for a second date right away. Even though we had met for the first time less than a month earlier, I still cared enough about her that I didn't want to lose her. I wanted another chance.

Before starting the car to take her home, I took a deep breath. "I'm sorry."

"About what?"

"The date. I feel like it was a bust."

"Why? I thought we had a good time."

I responded in the absolute worst way if I wanted that chance for a second date. "No, it didn't go as I planned. You see . . ." I fidgeted with my keys. *How do I say this without making her think I am deranged and need to be kept far away?*

Cindy turned to face me fully and took my hand. "What?"

"I believe God has told me we are to marry, and I didn't know what to do with that." I sat and held my breath.

She turned back and looked straight ahead. "Wow! I've never heard a line like that before." She paused. "I just don't know. I'll pray about it."

I let the air out of my lungs. *Well, she didn't run away screaming.* "Good. I like that. I mean, I couldn't have asked or expected anything more."

A few days later, I called to see if she would like to go on another date. To my surprise, she accepted.

Before we left for our date, we spent a little time with the family she was living with, the Pattons. I knew they were her temporary guardians, so I wanted them to know they could trust me.

The second date was followed by a third. We spent time together at the Drop-In meetings as well as at Sunday services. For three weeks we spent as much time together as we could.

When my birthday arrived near the end of March, I spent it with her just hanging out in my apartment. She caught me up on the latest happenings with her at school. By now many of her friends were also mine, so I enjoyed hearing her talk about them. In turn, I shared how things were going at work. Each day was becoming more difficult there with a boss who came to work smelling of beer. We ended up back at my apartment.

We had just settled on the couch when she turned and looked at me. "I hope you like my present for you."

I was puzzled, as I didn't see her bring anything in with her.

She handed me a card. I opened it and stared at the words, *I love you.*

It was now my turn to have emotions ricochet within my body. Those were the words I had longed to hear. I had held back saying them, choking on them. I refused to push my luck. Only three weeks had passed since our first date—the one I nearly bailed on, the one I made a total wreck of.

I continued staring at the card. Did she mean the life-partner-forever love? "It's wonderful. I've been wanting to say that to you, but I needed to hear you say it first. I love you too."

We sealed that moment with our first real kiss packed with all the love and commitment we could put into it.

The rest of our dates mainly consisted of talking, always getting to know each other's hearts more. Our discussions turned toward getting married. Our first choice was to elope. Neither wanted to be center stage. Nope. No fancy wedding for us. Now we just needed to tell her parents.

Cindy called and informed her mom, who answered, "Let me talk with Mrs. Patton."

Cindy and I sat holding hands, looking first at each other and then at Mrs. Patton, imagining what Cindy's mom was saying or asking. The speed of our courtship raised one big question, no doubt: did I get her pregnant?

Mrs. Patton handled that question for us. "Oh, absolutely not. I can guarantee it. Why, they even ask me to go with them on their dates."

When I heard that, I was so thankful we had taken the time to gain the family's trust.

We got the go-ahead from her parents, though her mom had the final word: "Have a church wedding. You can have anything you want. Just don't elope."

Wanting to develop a good relationship with her parents, whom I hadn't even met yet, we agreed.

That presented several problems for me, though. Lack of money loomed as one, but another tradition posed a greater snag: family photos. I wouldn't have Dad in our wedding photos, with us appearing as a happy family. If only he wouldn't come at all. I knew I had to invite him and that I couldn't shut him out of our lives completely (not that

I wanted to deep down), but some occasions required special finesse to produce perfect memories. Well, that was the reasoning I followed.

My problems with my boss at the clothing store worsened. He cut my hours so my only recourse was to quit and find a job that would pay more. I landed one back in my hometown of Salem as an assistant department store manager. Living an hour from Cindy forced our dates to be fewer and more targeted. We had less than two months to put the wedding plans together.

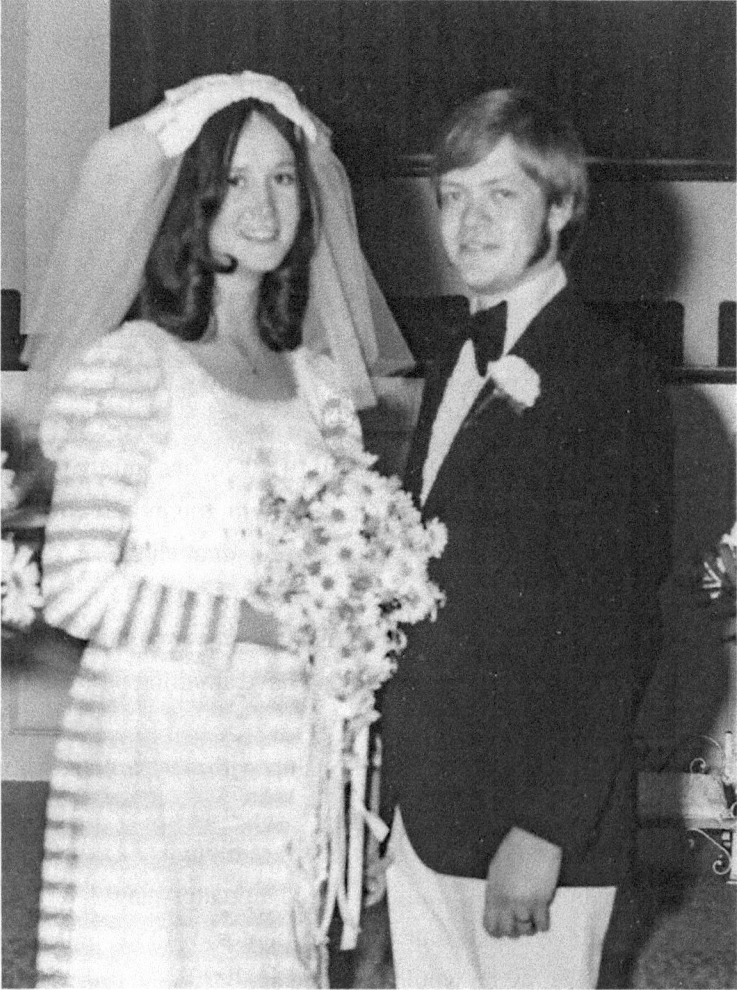

Cindy and I forty-nine years ago.

On August 10, 1973, six months after our first date, we got married in our church in Marion. And I didn't have to worry about Dad being in the photos. Though he attended the wedding, because of his stroke, going to the basement for the reception and cake cutting, then walking back up to the sanctuary for photos was too much for him. He stayed in the basement until it was time for us to drive off.

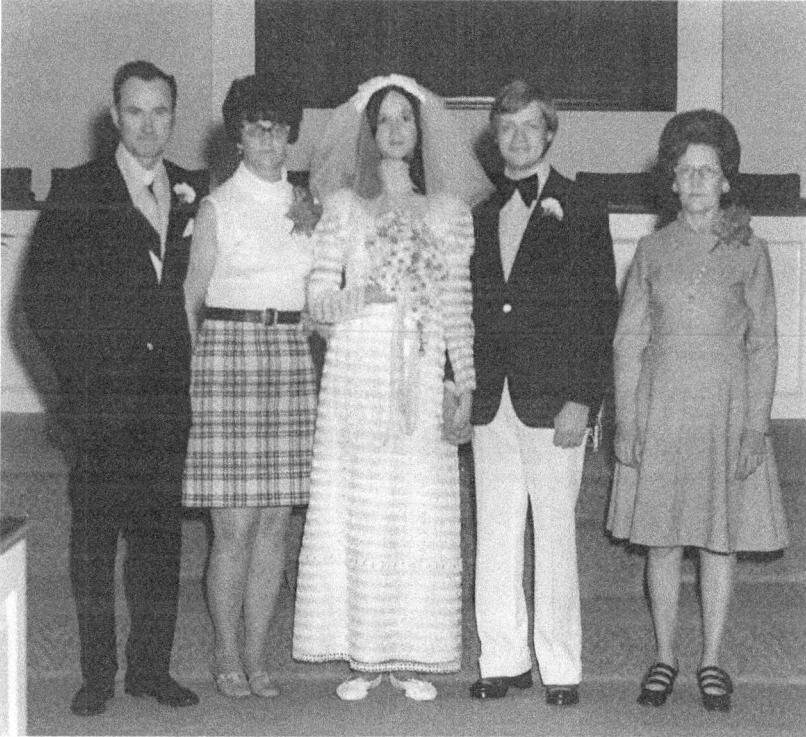

In early years, this group gave comfort—no Dad in it. Now it serves as a reminder of the cleansing and freedom Jesus has done.

My store manager gave me only the weekend off for our honeymoon. Between that and low finances, our time away was close to home and short. Sunday afternoon, we pulled into the driveway of our first nesting place back in my hometown of Salem. The rental cottage was about a block from my grandma Huff, and Cindy delighted walking down and spending time with her. She enjoyed getting to know, love, and appreciate all my family.

We were settling in quite nicely. Well, not financially, but we had hope. Then God spoke to my heart again. While what to expect wasn't clear, I sensed some sort of change coming. Cindy and I prayed about it, eventually talking with our pastor for any counsel he might have. He thought I would be well suited for something in Christian education, so I started looking into what Christian colleges had to offer.

I felt it only fair to inform the store manager of my plans to start back to college after the first of the year but that they included giving him and the store all I could for the Christmas rush and returns. I stalled as long as I could withstand the urge to tell him, finally caving the first week of December.

My boss, a Christian who attended church services regularly, would surely understand, I figured. He proved to be more practical than understanding. "If it is not your goal to be the manager of a store, I don't need you. You can leave now or work through to the end of the week."

Needing the money, I chose to work through the week, hoping the Lord would open a door for us or speak clear direction immediately. My meager salary did not allow us to get any money saved up.

I went home for lunch and told Cindy how it went with the manager. We spent most of the lunch hour praying. As I headed out the door to return to work, Cindy asked if she should call her parents.

I think my shoulders might have slumped in embarrassment, but I said, "We've been married only four months. They deserve to know what is happening with their daughter."

She made three calls that afternoon. Two went unanswered, followed by crying and more prayers. She was about to hang up on the third try when her dad answered. With a peaceful voice, Cindy explained why she called, adding, "We know Jesus is in control, so we are confident that everything will work out fine. We don't want you to worry, but Charley and I thought you should know."

A few minutes later, Cindy's dad called back, saying he had a job waiting for me in Aurora if I wanted it. When Cindy told me after I got home from work, I laughed with a sigh of relief. It seemed God was checking to see if I really meant it when I said He could be in control. For months I had rejected advice from Mom and one of Dad's cousins to find work in Aurora, saying the last place on earth I wanted to live was in a larger city like Aurora, Illinois. After our wedding, I told Cindy the last job on earth I wanted was a guard in the security company under her father.

Four months after our wedding, at the height of the Christmas season, Cindy and I moved four-and-a-half hours north to Aurora, where I worked as a security guard with her father as my supervisor. When we could afford it and my work schedule allowed, we drove back to Salem on weekends. Making sure we allotted time to visit Dad while we were there added pressure on our trips. For me, dropping in and saying hi fulfilled my duty, my obligation as a son to him. I struggled with wanting to build a relationship only to be disappointed again. He had crossed me too many times. But my renewed faith nudged me, despite my objections.

Cindy and Dad got along well. Somehow, she could interpret his wrong word or broken sentences and understand what he was trying to say. She would tease him and get him to laugh. I liked that. His laughter seldom erupted in my early years. Their fun together reignited hope in me, a hope that he would become a Christian, a hope that we could have some kind of father/son thing that would last. I started praying for his salvation again.

At the same time, memories of the years of physical and psychological wounds kept me from engaging him in the same way Cindy could. I still couldn't talk about Dad to others without anger and bitterness seeping out in what I said or how I related a story. So I tried to avoid the subject.

Two years after our marriage, our firstborn came into our lives. I called different family members to tell them our exciting news: we had a son. Dad was visiting Kenny and Phyllis when I called them, so Phyllis relayed my news to everyone. I heard some conversation in the background and waited for Phyllis to tell me what was said. "Your dad wants to know how his feet are."

I wasn't surprised by his question. After all, I had been born with clubfeet, and to be honest, that was the first thing I checked on my son. Add to that the standard his aunts held that Huffs should never marry because of the hereditary disabilities in our family. "Tell him they're perfect."

Phyllis relayed my answer. Returning to our conversation, she added, "He asked the same thing of us with each one of our children. I'm told he has asked about some of your cousins' kids too."

He asked again when my second son was born. He worried until he saw or was told the feet were normal, worried that they'd have feet like I had been born with.

In these days, Jesus began speaking to me that I needed to forgive Dad completely. I didn't like it, but I tried. I knew my attempts failed whenever I talked about my childhood memories and anger rose. These moments often sparked a response from Cindy.

"I don't remember you ever talking about that time with your dad."

I shrugged. "It never came up, I guess." That was a lie. I had not talked about it and many other clashes because I chose to seal them up, hoping they would die in dark recesses of my heart.

It was around that time when the Lord introduced me to the most remarkable man I'd ever known. Bob Sadler. The Spirit of the Lord so anointed him you could feel it. Having been asked to run the sound and recording equipment, I always arrived at church early and got everything set up. One Sunday morning, after completing the setup, I felt love wash over the room like a giant wave. I turned to Cindy. "Who just came in?"

"I don't know. Why?"

"Something just happened. I felt it."

I craned my neck but could see no one special. Too many people were standing and milling about between the front of the church where I was and the entrance, blocking my view of the doorway.

Several people moved to gather around someone. I was right about what I felt. Someone special had come in. I stood and then could see Bob, an African American born in South Carolina in 1911, and he was greeting people. He came to be the special speaker at our church that week, sharing through music, testimonies, and teaching, his message of freedom through forgiveness.

Cindy and I knew a bit of his life story, and his love never ceased to amaze us. He had every reason imaginable to be filled with mistrust and hatred. When he was five years old, his dad sold him and two older sisters to a local plantation owner as slaves—fifty-one years after the Civil War had officially ended slavery. One sister died from infections caused by being poked with a hot iron. The plantation owner and some of his friends had been drinking too much and thought it fun to see her jump and squeal. Unable to look at her and her injuries, he sent her out from being a house slave to working in the cotton fields.

As a teenager, Bob escaped from the plantation and made it to the north where he learned to read and play piano. Later, Jesus became his Savior, Lord, and Master. His heart changed so completely that he returned to his former owner who was a broken, old man to witness to him about the amazing love of Jesus.

Bob had not been given a middle name at birth. To express his love and complete freedom from hatred, he took the plantation owner's family name as his middle name and became Robert Dean Sadler. Because of Jesus' love, Bob had overcome bitterness and any thoughts of retribution.

Meeting his dad years later, Bob asked why he'd sold them.

Tears came to his father's eyes as he said, "So I could buy a bottle of whiskey."

At first, Bob couldn't believe their lives were worth so little to him, but he reached over and forgave him.[1]

I wanted that kind of love to wash away the bitterness I still had in my heart. But I wasn't sure Dad and I could ever get to that place—not even too sure if I *could* forgive him. I tried to imagine what it would be like if it happened. Naturally, he would see how much he had wronged Mom and me and would come to me and ask for forgiveness. That was the right way. After all, he was the perpetrator; I was the victim. I would cry when he asked for forgiveness. I knew I would because tears flowed even as I imagined it. Then maybe Dad would go to church with me, as had been my desire from my youth.

My mind created beautiful scenes and various ways it would unfold. But the one thing missing that I never focused on was how I would forgive him after his apology. It seemed to be implied, but I put less emphasis on my forgiving than on his asking.

Soon after hearing Bob's testimony at our church, Jesus gave me another strong nudge. Cindy and I were reading *Tramp for the Lord* together. We sat with our cups of tea, settled in our comfy chairs, and took turns reading—sometimes choking with tears as we read of the tragedies and trials Corrie ten Boom had endured.

In this book Corrie, who had lived through being a prisoner in a concentration camp during World War II, shared an account of a former prison guard—one she remembered who had taken extra pleasure in inflicting pain and cruelty—extending his hand to her several years later and asking forgiveness.

I read the words and didn't doubt her testimony, but I still questioned, *How could she?* I knew what I went through was a picnic compared to her experience, but I also knew the pain and depth of bitterness in my heart toward my dad. To my question of how, I added why. When Dad hadn't asked for forgiveness nor expressed any remorse, why should I forgive him? But the Spirit began to nudge me. Again, in obedience to the Spirit's prompting, I tried.

Dad occasionally got different family members to help him get on a bus or plane to Chicago, where we would pick him up. In each of our week-long visits with Dad, I went out of my way to help him feel welcome and comfortable in our home. He went to church with us once and took us out to dinner afterward. He refused to go ever again, but he would still take us out to dinner after we came home from the service. From the outside, we looked like a normal, healthy family. He took Cindy's teasing well and even accepted hugs from her. I saw hints of the beginnings of a family bond, but in private moments, little things pushed the seething soul within me out into the open.

My inner cauldron boiled over after one of Dad's visits didn't end well. On the day of his flight home, Cindy, our two boys, Dad, and I loaded into the car for the airport. I dropped him with Cindy and Nathan, our eldest, at the departure gate, then parked the car in the terminal garage, keeping our youngest with me.

After our goodbyes, we got back into the car and merged into the heavy traffic, leaving the airport. I

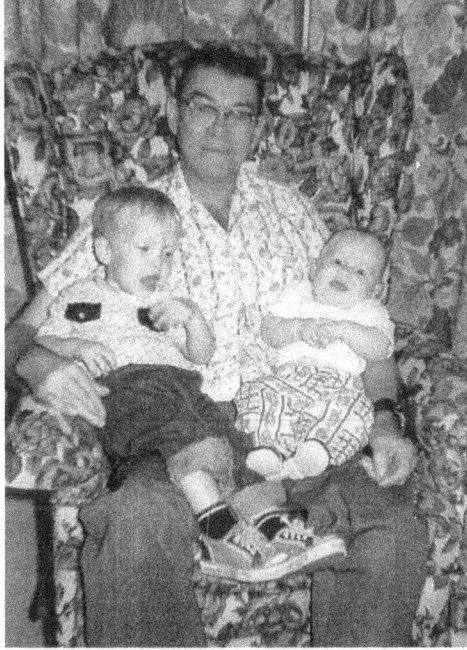

Dad enjoying our sons 1977

didn't have to look. I knew Cindy had her eyes locked on me, studying me. I checked my rearview mirrors. I hated Chicago traffic, especially from O'Hare Airport.

Don't say a word, Cindy. I don't want to talk. The deadly silence battled the turbulent emotions choking me. *Forty more minutes to home. Can I make it?*

"Charley, are you mad at me?"

I checked the mirrors again. A car zigzagged between lanes. *I better keep an eye on him. He's an accident ready to happen.* I stayed clear of him.

"Well, are you?"

I exhaled. "We need to talk."

"You didn't answer my question."

Can't we not talk now so I can think? I stuffed my emotions, forcing my words to come out gently. "Yes. And no."

"What does that mean?"

"It means I have too many thoughts racing through my mind to make any sense of them. But first, I need to get us through this crazy traffic and home safely. I would appreciate it if we didn't talk now."

Cindy turned on some music to entertain our two young boys in the back seat and to swallow the silence between us. I wished I could snap my fingers and be home, away from the traffic, the noise, and the prying eyes. Most of all, I wanted to be free from the mayhem in my mind.

In my solitude, I rehearsed the events and conversations we'd had during the week. Overall, Dad's visit had been good. We'd succeeded in being more than civil to each other. Dad seemed more at ease during our time together—not demanding any special treatment. He even honored Cindy's rule of no smoking in the house and went outside to smoke without complaining. So why were my emotions boiling? Before I could sort out one thought and find its resolution, we pulled into our driveway. On autopilot, I helped Cindy get the boys into the house and ready to go play.

I still didn't know where to start our conversation. I was standing in our house with no traffic to fight. Shouldn't that have calmed me and given me clarity? It failed.

And Cindy stood in front of me, waiting for me to speak. The first question in my mind—perhaps the most menacing one that stood between us—burst out at her. "How can you be so nice to him?"

"How can I what?"

"After the hell he made Mom and me live in, how can you be so nice to him?"

"Because I have never seen him as you remember him. I see him only as a man seriously crippled by a stroke. He needs help, understanding, compassion, and family."

"He doesn't deserve family. He wasn't there when we needed it."

"Don't make me hate him."

Her words slapped me into a new awareness. I sighed, feeling my anger quickly dissipate. "No. . . . Of course I don't want you to hate him. It's just . . ." I paused, searching for the right words. "Let me put it this way. If it weren't for the boys, I don't know if I would let him in our lives now. If you haven't guessed, I've been selective in sharing bits of my past because I didn't want to control how you looked at Dad. I may have made a wrong choice. Your approach to him is a world apart from mine. That difference is what I am having trouble with. I think I need to let you know more about my past. We need to have a united point of reference in how we let Dad into our family."

Cindy took my hand. "If it will make you feel better."

As memories surfaced, puddles formed on my bottom eyelids, waiting for a blink to splash them.

Cindy pulled me close, wrapped her arms around me, and laid my head on her shoulder. "Poor Charley."

CHAPTER 9

THE LONG-AWAITED MIRACLE

I am going to heal your dad. First I will heal his heart toward me and then I will heal his body.

Those were the words Jesus spoke into my heart days before Cindy and I married. They were what I returned to with each step toward being able to love Dad. Those words bolstered my sagging confidence when each passing year brought little or no change in him. That hope helped me move from tolerance to cordiality to genuine affection toward my father.

And yet changes in Dad were not happening—at least not the changes I wanted to see in my time frame. He should have been meeting me at that elusive half-way mark. If I showed him honor and respect, shouldn't I see gratitude and favor in return? But Dad's emotional bank accepted deposits with limited if any withdrawals. I wasn't expecting him to show fatherly love because I didn't think he knew how, but that didn't stop me from craving it. Not having his love because of his drunken condition, I understood. His wait-and-see attitude toward my overtures perhaps cut me deeper than his moments of rage. I knew unfulfilled expectations fueled my irritation toward the love Cindy gave him, a love that, in my eyes, covered or ignored all the wrong he had done to me.

After the ride home from dropping Dad at the airport, I could say for the first time what festered in my heart. I told her I loved her, but I felt so hurt by her when she loved my abuser the way she did. I tried to keep from letting my pent-up anger out on her, but how could I sweetly give someone poison? I looked into Cindy's eyes and saw tears fighting to squeeze out. She'd appealed to me to not make her stop showing him love.

Cindy's request cut me deeply, but in a good way. It severed the cords of self-pity and bitterness I had allowed to ensnare me. In that moment of freedom, the Holy Spirit showed me what He was trying to do in and for me. As the proverb says, "Faithful are the wounds of a friend" (Proverbs 27:6, NKJV). Jesus was so faithful to me to bring truths from His Word to help me in my time of need.

In Cindy's prayer for me following her tearful appeal, she spoke of my kindness and compassion toward Dad one minute and my seething bitterness the next. She knew in her spirit about the battle taking place in my heart.

Through the months and years that followed, she watched my acts of kindness toward him go unrewarded. Even her best suggestions of what we could do with and for Dad seemed to do little or nothing against the wall he had built up. She could see the sincerity in my efforts and prayed more for me. At the same time, she knew I still had deep-seated anger toward him. She carried our efforts of love as far as we could take them, and she wooed me back from my trails of bitter revenge.

I still demanded that Dad make amends, that he apologize, that he confess to the reign of terror I'd lived through at his hands. But the Holy Spirit continued to nudge me to forgive him anyway.

One such Spirit push came to me in the form of a long-play vinyl record (LP). A friend was thinning his collection and thought I would like a Kenneth Copeland album he had. One song on the LP moved me to tears every time I listened to it. The song, "I Have Returned," dripped with pathos and nostalgia. It recalled the stories of Bible heroes and put the singer's personal heroes (mother and father) beside them. One stanza spoke of learning who Jesus is while sitting and listening to his mother. Memories of those times Mom and I studied the Sunday school lessons together flooded my mind at those words.

Between the times Mom and I studied together and when I received this recording, my life went through very dark days. The lyrics spoke to me about how—through it all—the Lord never gave up on me. Joy welled up and spilled out my eyes.

As I learned the words, I sang along with the record until the next stanza. The lyrics refer to the father who reflected God's goodness. That was so far from my experience. I wouldn't sing those words. I couldn't. It would be a lie and a hypocrisy to do so. But deep within, I wanted it to be so.

Lack of forgiveness sat like a boulder on my chest, pinning the childlike heart beneath it. My efforts to forgive Dad on my own flatlined. My love was weak. When the memories of the pain and fear from my childhood and teen years arose, they took over my emotions. This evidence revealed I still held onto unforgiveness toward Dad.

Good times with Dad became better and more frequent. A sense of normal relations settled in, only to have a conversation bring up the past and cast me back to my starting point. I had in my heart a long scroll of Dad's offenses needing to be reconciled. I tried to forgive him of all of them as one packaged deal, but that didn't work for me. Forgotten memories would capture my attention at unwanted times and throw me into the pain and rejection and bitterness that I thought I had overcome.

In my private conversations with God, I asked Him to remove the barriers in my life hindering the healing. I rehearsed verses of promises that spoke to my prayers, hoping my faith would be built up if it had been found lacking. *Why, God? Why am I still stuck? Dad's time is surely getting shorter. Another stroke will probably kill him. What is blocking the changes I seek?*

God's answer to me came in an unexpected and especially unwanted way. This time Jesus didn't tell me to forgive Dad, He told me to ask Dad to forgive *me*.

"What? No way! I'm the victim here, God!"

My heart hardened and closed to the idea. Jesus reminded me He had also been the victim. Sinless, He hung in agony on the cross and from it forgave those who put Him there. Not only had they not asked for it, but they were still hurling insults and spitting on Him as Jesus forgave them. I realized my sin put me among those who yelled, "Crucify Him!" until the day came when I asked Jesus to forgive me. A crack formed in my wall against the Holy Spirit's prompting.

My memories kept locking me into a victim's pity party. Then Jesus pitted my emotional and physical pain against Dad's eternity.

What if your dad is looking at what a Christian is like through your example? Would he want anything to do with it?

I thought about the nearly three decades I had spent wanting Dad to change. Could my behavior, while claiming to be a Christian, have been a hindrance? The weight of that possibility buried me in a wave of guilt and remorse. Had God been working in Dad's heart, but my impatience worked against what God was doing? Jesus reminded me of His love for Dad and of some instances when He had given Dad special opportunities to receive forgiveness and salvation.

Besides having different family members who reached out to him with gifts, prayers, and words, Dad had other God-arranged encounters. When I needed it most, God reminded me of one forgotten event after another.

Details of one day when I was a young teenager played out in my mind almost like a video. Dad had unpredictably come straight home from work without stopping at the bar. He didn't say much at first, but after dinner he asked if Mom or I knew a dwarf.

I sat quiet, not knowing if I was really to be part of the conversation. Mom continued clearing the dishes from the table. "Yes, why?"

"I pulled into a truck stop to fill up on gas. While I was checking the tires and the chains holding my haul in place, this dwarf walked over to me from his camper. He said he noticed the name on the truck said it was from Salem, Illinois, and wanted to know if I was from Salem."

I wondered if this was the man who helped when I was nine to know who Jesus was. Every nerve cluster in my body fired like miniature firecrackers. I sat on my hands to keep them from going wild in anticipation of the possibilities. Dad didn't seem to notice.

Mom wanted to hear the whole story. "What did he have to say after that?"

"He went on to talk about singing at a gospel crusade in one of the churches there a few years ago."

It was Lowell Mason! Who else could it have been? The song evangelist met my dad at a truck stop to share the love of Jesus with Dad. How did that happen? Unbelievable. Yet that amazing encounter took place. The way Dad talked about it, I could tell it had some kind of impact on him. The tremble in his voice. The level of detail. He talked about Lowell in ways I had never heard him speak of any other man.

I wept as Jesus brought this and other memories up. I shared these thoughts with Cindy, and we prayed. I promised the Lord I would ask Dad to forgive me.

Dad never came up frequently, maybe twice a year, so a few months passed before we picked him up at the airport again. A little time into that visit, I asked Cindy to be praying. I had decided then was the time to ask Dad to forgive me. I needed the Lord's help. I didn't know how to begin. Does anyone know how to start a conversation like this? The silence between us became unbearable—much more uncomfortable than saying what I had practiced.

"Dad, Jesus has been speaking to me about how I have been a poor example to you of what it is to be a Christian. He has shown me how I have been a stubborn, rebellious son, not respecting you as I should. I need to ask you if you will forgive me."

Blurting it out the way I did may have made it sound insincere and memorized, but I had to get it out. I looked at him for any reaction.

"'Bout time." He didn't blink an eye. No signs of melting or remorse. If his face spoke anything, it spoke of justification.

I hadn't practiced for that response and let out a nervous chuckle. "It's not like you made it easy for me."

The lingering effects of his stroke made themselves apparent as he struggled with his response. "D-d-didn't. Have. To."

Okay, that retort stung. I stiffened and answered him in kind. "You didn't have to make it so hard either."

Dad's expression still didn't change. He looked satisfied, as if he had just won the contest.

Had the stroke erased his memories of my growing up years or was this more of his obstinance? "Dad, you used to beat me black and blue. You threatened Mom and me with your shotgun and nearly killed us many times when you insisted on driving, even though you were too drunk. We lived in constant fear. My worst behavior was still better than much of your good. Don't you think I deserve an apology?"

Dad's "'Bout time" response had triggered my pain reaction again. I don't remember the rest of our conversation. I know only that my badgering an apology out of him destroyed what God was prepared to do.

The glaring truth at the moment was how I had blown it again. I had entered our conversation with Jesus at my side and His words in my mouth. I knew in advance Dad might not be open to my apology. His response struck me as if he put all the problem on me. I felt I had to set the record straight. I pushed for what I wanted—Dad accepting responsibility for his actions.

I needed to be humbled more. For the next two-plus years, Jesus worked on me. He showed me the times I had rejected Dad as anything more than my biological father and had done my own things over his objections. Like the one afternoon I wanted to go into town to meet up with some friends where one worked. Dad told me to stay home. I viewed it as another example of his wanting to control. "I'm not needed here, and I see no reason why you should have any say."

"If that car leaves the garage, I'll show you I have a say."

"It's my car. I pay for the gas and repairs."

"If you're going to town, you will have to walk. That's how it's going to be."

"Fine."

So I did. I trimmed off some of the five-plus miles to town by walking along the railroad tracks and made it to my destination before the dark storm clouds rolling in from the west released their fury on me. They caught up with me and seemed to hang above my head like those thought bubbles over a cartoon character.

Jesus brought many such memories to mind during those two years. Helping me relive past events with fresh eyes, Jesus used them to work out in me what I couldn't see by myself. The conversations Jesus, Cindy, and I had about them became the foundation for my efforts to convince Dad my apology was sincere. My stone heart softened more, and genuine love—and real forgiveness—took root and grew.

Little changes in Dad's responses around us gave Cindy and me hope. Dad started letting us hug him hello and goodbye. He would respond to us with, "I love. You. Too." He even started holding hands with us when we prayed a blessing over our meals. But in every other way, he continued to resist the grace Jesus had for him.

In December 1978, a biopsy confirmed Dad had cancer in his lungs and lymph nodes. The doctors gave him three to six months to live. Treatment would likely extend his life only three months. Kenny went with me to bring Dad home from the hospital after having the testing done. My older brother—the strong one, the one closer to Dad—put me into the back of the van with Dad for the trip home. He confused me by doing that. It made more sense to me that he should be the one to tell Dad what the doctor said about the tests. After all, he had made Dad proud. He drank and smoked with Dad. They had shared times hunting, fishing, and playing baseball. It all added up to one conclusion in my mind, but Kenny couldn't do it. Kenny set me up to tell our father.

As Dad lay on the ambulance gurnee, he looked straight ahead and finally broke the silence. "What d—doctor say?"

"No one told you?" I was stalling.

"No."

I cleared my throat and sat forward in the seat. "Well, the biopsy proved to be cancer. The doctor said it has spread, and he gave you three to six months to live without any treatment. Treatment might add three months."

A few tears rolled down Dad's cheeks, then silence enveloped us again.

I didn't know how long he would remember what I had just told him. Even nine years after his stroke, Dad often forgot words or said wrong words. Sometimes he would forget every part of what he intended to say. I thought maybe this was the God-ordained time for Dad to break his resistance against the Lord. Facing eternity with such harsh news clearly had his attention. I tried talking with him about being ready to see Jesus face-to-face, but my words seem to bounce off him. Dad still wasn't ready to surrender his heart and what remained of his life to Jesus.

For the next three months, I drove the four-and-a-half hours down to Salem on weekends to be with Dad. I counted it a big effort and sacrifice on my part. For the six years we lived in Aurora, I never traveled after Thanksgiving and didn't venture far until Easter or later. The weather in northern and central Illinois could swoop in and make safe driving impossible. I never thought traveling during those months was worth taking a chance. But a chance is all I had left for Dad. I reminded the Lord how certain I was about a promise for Dad's salvation. That promise included healing. His healing didn't matter so much to me anymore. I had one top priority: to know he would stand before God forgiven. That consumed my thoughts and prayers.

Cindy and I prayed each time I left for Salem that I could share my faith in a way Dad would receive. And every time my report back to Cindy ended with, "No one ever gave me a chance to talk with Dad alone."

Even Grandma would hobble over to the table where Dad and I were sitting to listen to our conversations. One of those times revealed something I never knew about my dad. All our lives, Dad insisted animals should never be in a house. They were made to live outside, no exceptions. Grandma let it slip that Dad had a dog that slept with him when he was a boy. None of his brothers or sisters enjoyed such a privilege.

I looked across at Dad and shouted with shock mixed with laughter, "What?"

Dad's face reddened with an embarrassed chuckle. He never explained why he changed his stand on this matter for his own house.

I could tell his time was running out. He was visibly weaker with each trip down. Cindy and I changed our prayer focus and began praying that anyone having contact with Dad would be a Christian with a heart for sharing the gospel. Days passed like the second hand on a clock. We enlisted friends to pray with us. Each trip revealed Dad's cancer racing to a quick end. Every weekend I returned home frustrated that my aunts and uncles never let me have time alone with him. I wondered what they were afraid of. I never thought that perhaps they could be as anxious as I was over Dad's salvation and also wanted to hear the moment he repented. I kept my words locked up for a one-on-one with him.

During these weeks, Uncle Bob and I talked often on the phone. He told me Dad had his funeral and all arrangements detailed and paid. One detail included who would preach his funeral. Dad had remembered a man who had worked with him at the tank company. The man had met Jesus in a dramatic way and left the company to become a pastor.

Hope within Cindy and me leaped with joy to hear this. It sounded like the divine appointment made in heaven for this time and place. Dad evidently saw something in this man's life years earlier that still had influence on him. We imagined how this was going to work out between Dad and his friend. The next call dropped us hard. Dad wouldn't respond to his friend's testimony and challenge. We prayed harder.

Days later, Dad's water heater broke. A repairman responded to a call, checked it out, replaced it, and then sat down and shared his faith with Dad. Uncle Bob said Dad prayed with the man and accepted Jesus as his savior, assuring me that it was real.

What made the difference? Was it something the repairman said? How could a complete stranger have a stronger witness than an old friend whose changed life Dad had seen? I don't know why God chose him above all the others in Dad's life. This I do know: God had a perfect plan all along. I cautiously rejoiced at the news, still wanting to know for sure for myself.

On the drive downstate the next weekend, I wrestled with my doubts. I knew of too many who found Jesus in the middle of crisis but forgot Him when the crisis passed. Foxhole Christians, they are called.

"Jesus, I thank You for this word of hope. If I'm to believe it, then You've answered our prayers. But how will I know?" I cried out. "I need to know it's genuine. Does Dad really know You? What do I say or ask him?"

Then a voice in my heart spoke clearly. *Ask him if he loves Me.*

"Lord, that's too simple. Isn't it?"

"Just ask him if he loves Me."

Tears flooded down my face. I nearly had to pull off the road as my vision became blurred. When I could see clearly again, I resumed highway speed. My prayers took on a new focus. Thankfulness. I kept exhorting myself to ask Dad if he loved Jesus and then drop it. God's word to me was very specific. I didn't want to repeat my earlier mistakes.

The rest of the drive seemed over early. Uncle Bob, Aunt Ruby, and Grandma were there with Dad. A prayer whispered through my mind, *Jesus, give me time with Dad that I need.*

Hospice had brought in a hospital bed for Dad. He appeared to be sleeping, so I sat at the table with the family to talk. They updated me on how he was doing. *Why did you wait so long, Dad? The end doesn't have to be like this.*

A rustle from Dad's direction got my attention. A glance toward him confirmed he was looking at us. I moved my chair beside him and leaned in close so we could talk privately. In the background, the others continued their conversation. I was alone with Dad for the first time since the ride home from the hospital three months ago.

"Dad, you are about to take your last road trip. Are you ready?"

"Yes."

"I need to ask you a question, Dad." I paused and took in his tired and worn face. "Do you love Jesus?"

He locked eyes with mine with an intensity but without malice I had never seen before. "Yes."

I know I've made this mistake before, Lord, but forgive me. I have to ask him more. "Did you ask Jesus into your heart?"

Again, that look. It couldn't have been more intense even if he had held my face immovable in his hands, forcing me to look at him. "Yes."

I fought back the tears—tears of joy, and tears of repentance for disobeying the Lord. *Why couldn't I just believe?* I had asked God to tell me how I would know for sure. He answered me, but it wasn't good enough for me. *Heal my unbelieving heart, Lord.*

Then Dad locked eyes with me again and without hesitation or struggle with words he added, "I only wish I knew the Bible as well as you do."

I gasped at his words and how they flowed. "Soon, Dad, you will know it better than me. To all the questions anyone has ever had, you will know the answers."

Grandma stood and limped toward the bed to stand near us. She blew her nose on an already well used tissue. "He was my champion."

"How so, Grandma?" I thought of the Dark Ages and the way they used the word *champion* and wondered if she meant it in that way—a shining knight to the rescue.

"He was always the strong one. But for his smoking and drinking, he was healthier than the rest. I tried to get him to stop those things, but . . ." She wiped her nose again. Her face showed what she held in her heart but couldn't speak. Grandma had been a widow twenty-three years and now she would see one of her children buried too. She had always said she wanted to live to be one hundred years old. At age eighty-nine, she was well on her way. I didn't think she considered making it to one hundred might include outliving any of her children. I reached over and gave her hand a gentle squeeze.

As I left Salem that weekend, I couldn't wait to share with everyone back in Aurora what Jesus had done on this trip. My words flowed out as soon as I stepped into our house, trying hard to make sure I remembered to tell everything. Cindy peppered me with questions, asking for more details. I hadn't finished answering them when the phone rang.

The voice on the other end of the call sang with excitement. Gayle, one of our prayer warriors, waited to call us until she was sure I would be home. "As I was praying on Saturday, I sensed the burden lift. Jesus spoke to my heart that I didn't need to pray for his salvation anymore."

She rejoiced with me as I shared what had happened, and we thanked the Lord for confirming His work.

In the days after that weekend, phone calls from Uncle Bob became more frequent as Dad's condition worsened daily. Before I could get back for another visit, I received the inevitable call. At first, I was glad the waiting was over and relieved that Dad's suffering was done. I remembered my last visit with him and became overcome with sorrow. After twenty-nine years of wanting to know Dad's love and approval, that brief moment with Dad as my brother in Christ was all I got?

Uncle Bob, who was Dad's executor, had continued talking and shared Dad's final moments while I was lost in my thoughts. Just when I tuned back into what he was saying, he shifted the conversation to practical matters. "The funeral home is very busy this week, so we had to fit into a schedule. I hope you don't mind, but we scheduled the funeral to be on your birthday. Do you have a problem with that? We can delay it if it would really bother you."

I considered the irony of the timing. Dad wasn't at my birth, but on its anniversary, we were burying his body. I remembered Dot—my friend's mother, my shelter during my teens—telling me she nearly killed herself when her second child was born. She refused to let him be born on the day her brother had died. Would my birthdays forever have a cloud over them because of this? Why would they? One of the greatest things I'd desired all my life had happened. Dad knew Jesus and was with Him. I had no doubt that truth would add to the celebration. "No. No problem."

Uncle Bob let out a sigh. "I am so glad you weren't here to see him. His body swelled up. His head became the size of a basketball. He looked more like a monster than human. I'm grateful you were spared seeing that."

Those words echoed in my mind as I prepared to attend Dad's funeral. I learned it would be an open casket. What was I going to see?

I walked into the funeral home the evening of the wake and looked toward the casket. *I thank You, God, for doing what You promised in Dad's salvation. But where is his healing?*

Closest family members had already arrived. I nodded to each one who looked my way. Grandma was sitting in an overstuffed chair placed in the front row for her.

As I walked to the front of the room where Dad's body lay and stood beside him, my breath caught in my throat. He looked twenty years younger and as if he had never been sick a single day.

Another scene from *The Hiding Place* flashed in my mind. Corrie ten Boom was captive in one of Germany's prison camps during World War II. She had seen her sister Betsy in the camp hospital and described her as bones with yellowed skin stretched tight over them— a grotesque marble statue yellowed with age. When Betsy died, a fellow inmate insisted Corrie go to the morgue to see her sister again. Corrie resisted. She knew the inhumane treatment of the Germans, but she finally gave in to an inmate's persistent nagging. Looking in the window at the morgue, Corrie could not believe what she saw. Betsy lay there looking like she did before the war started and as though angels had been combing her hair.

Yes, Lord, I see it. You healed Dad. You kept Your promise. It wasn't the way I thought it would be, but I thank You.

After the funeral, Uncle Bob said he had been carrying a secret for years. "Junior drank a little now and then when he was younger. He came home from the war (World War II) a heavy drinker. So listen to me when I tell you the war changed him. Dad made me swear I would not tell anyone what I'm about to tell you, but since everyone is dead that the secret would hurt, I think it's okay for me to tell you now."

Though I had no clue what he was talking about, I was intrigued.

"When my dad—your grandpa—was still alive, he would hear that your dad was in the tavern and not going home. Dad would go into the tavern to try to get Junior to go home. He told Junior he had drunk enough. Told him it was time for him to go home to Norma and the boys. Junior told Dad, 'I'm afraid to. The reason I stay and drink is I'm afraid of what I might do. There are times I feel like I could kill them and not be a bit sorry for it.'"

The image of the gun cabinet flashed in my mind. I shook it off, not wanting to miss anything Uncle Bob was saying.

"Your dad's drinking got worse after your grandpa died. I tried going into the tavern a few times like Dad had, but I didn't have the same influence over him Dad did, so I quit trying. Really hear me when I say, Charles, the war changed your dad."

I lived in an era when men were men. They handled their own problems. Family intervention nights never happened. Apparently, even when they knew murder was in the heart. In all those years of praying for a sober dad, I thought the monster Dad unleashed came to him through the beer he drank. The thought of the demons of murder being resident in him all the time never occurred to me. A question formed in my heart. Was it possible for dad to have been a greater danger sober than drunk?

I needed to see Dad through different eyes. *Jesus, heal me. Heal my memories.*

CHAPTER 10

PAINFUL, BLESSED HEALING

In the days after the funeral, I pondered what had happened in the previous two weeks. I couldn't shed a tear at the funeral because I knew Dad had settled into his new home in glory with Jesus. The service honored Jesus as much as it spoke of Dad's life and the people who loved him. I was glad I felt a member of that group—all because of what Jesus had done in me.

And yet at home the week after the funeral, my emotions started swinging and twirling like a carnival ride. It was usually when my thoughts stuck on the question why. Why had my lifetime of prayer been answered with those few minutes I had to enjoy Dad as my brother in Christ? Then I remembered Dad's surprising last words to me, spoken without any signs of the stroke he suffered. The monster who had wanted to beat me for being baptized affirmed I had chosen the right path and wanted to be more like me. Memories and the emotions tied to them would not leave me in that joyful place.

Even though Dad and I came to a point of reconciliation, complete with a blessing spoken over me, and even though my abuser was now dead and could never disappoint or harm me again, neither the freedom I received nor my new relationship with my dad was complete. In a general, big-picture sort of way, I had forgiven Dad. But I still experienced times when topics of conversation stirred scenes from my past, causing painful memories to erupt and emotions to burst within me. I had to forgive Dad for each of those memories every time they came up.

I tried to bury the past along with Dad and, more to the point, pack and store away his last words to me, but time proved that wasn't God's way. God wasn't done with me. I had asked Him to heal my memories. Being a faithful God, He set things in motion to answer that prayer.

And God uses anything and anyone at his disposal to accomplish His purposes. In more recent times, He chose to use one of our five children—my dog-groomer daughter Nicole—to give me understanding of how Jesus was answering my prayer for healing. She taught me that a dog can look all brushed and neat but still have a tangled mess in an undercoat. Sometimes, if the dog will be patient, the groomer or owner can work out all the knotted hair. Other times, the tangles can be so bad that the only solution is to shave the dog. Either way, detangling and shaving can be painful for the dog, though doing it is imperative. My life has been like those dogs. I have been able to present a good appearance to others—especially to those outside the family. They get to see my best image and not the tangled mess underneath layers of disguise. (I must have unconsciously learned that skill from my dad.)

For nearly forty years, God has been carefully untangling and combing out what I'd held concealed. As He has done this, He has given me an evolving understanding and image of my dad. My past is what it is. It hasn't changed or been rewritten, but Jesus has changed the way I look at Dad and has released me from being a victim still.

I hate that word *victim*—not only because I was one. I hate that abusers exist, creating victims. I hate that the word *victim* speaks of someone caught in some attack by another—whether physical, financial, or emotional—and who believes they are impotent to prevent or fight off the attack. I wanted to believe I had, over time, risen above my circumstances, but each emotional trigger proved I hadn't. When the MeToo movement started, I watched its progress with mixed emotions. My first reaction applauded the success of bringing such heinous wrongs to light, but I was also leery of it, perhaps because I realized I was an unwilling member of it. As the movement's momentum exploded, I saw their efforts for justice as holding no promise of total freedom from being labeled a victim. Their focus from the beginning was to see justice meted out on their abusers, hoping it would bring them closure.

I learned through my experiences that anything done to my abuser did nothing toward removing my victim tag. Instead, a bit of freedom came each time Jesus brought up a painful memory that by His grace I could forgive. The power of that truth became evident in 2018 when Cindy and I went to see the movie *I Can Only Imagine*. The movie is based on Bart Millard's life. Bart, a member of MercyMe and the lyric writer/composer of the song "I Can Only Imagine," had a life similar to my formative years.

Several scenes perfectly mirrored my own experiences with my alcoholic father. Seeing them portrayed on the big screen was more than I was prepared to sit through. In the darkened theater, I had a PTSD moment. I gripped Cindy's hand, trying not to squeeze too hard as tears flowed and my body shook. I forced myself to stay through the entire movie, knowing the outcome was good—in the life story portrayed and in my own circumstances, but the pain those scenes brought was very real.

A few years earlier, I had heard how several World War II veterans suffered after watching *Saving Private Ryan* and Vietnam veterans had relapses after watching *We Were Soldiers*, but I had difficulty understanding how or why. Until it happened to me.

That experience prompted me to look back over the years since Dad died and piece the memories together. Through the review process, I could see and understand what the Lord had been doing and could marvel at what He *has* done.

My change began with old, familiar verses taking on new meanings for me, new highlights on passages I had glossed over. In the sample prayer Jesus taught His disciples, He included, "Forgive us our debts [trespasses] as we forgive our debtors [those who trespass against us]" (Matthew 6:12). When Jesus first impressed upon me to forgive Dad, I had exempted Dad from those we should forgive. His actions were not a misunderstanding or simple missteps. His were blatant choices. Beatings and attempted murder didn't count in my mind. When the Holy Spirit spotlighted that verse for me, I saw that little word *as* and questioned its meaning and application. Had I been reciting and sometimes praying that God would forgive me *when* I forgive or *in the same measure* that I forgive others?

I rejected the idea because all was forgiven me on the cross, right?

The Holy Spirit then took me to other verses. Immediately following the Lord's example prayer, He added, "If you forgive men their trespasses, your heavenly Father will also forgive you. But if you do not forgive men their trespasses, neither will your Father forgive your trespasses" (Matthew 6:14-15). I pushed that verse away from me. I insisted Dad must apologize to me. I knew I would have to submit to that verse when he did, but my attitude was, *Yeah, like that is ever going to happen.*

While I don't believe Jesus was speaking about the forgiveness in salvation, I do see a truth that many don't want to admit. We can counteract our pleas for mercy if we insist on others getting what's coming to them. Or at least what we want coming to them. I was trying my best to be a good son to Dad in his final years. I believed I meant it when I said I forgave him. But little reminders could trigger the pain I still had festering within me. In those moments, I wanted Dad to experience the suffering I had endured and still carried with me.

At the time, I likened God's process in me to treating an infection under a scab. I knew I needed to endure the pain of having the scab pulled off and a disinfectant applied so my wounds could heal from the inside out. Without that, the infection could spread and become spiritually fatal. I resisted at first. I wanted justice to fall upon Dad and mercy upon me. The Holy Spirit showed me that if I didn't forgive, then my pride and arrogance—my stepping into the Lord's place as judge—kept my sin attached to me, keeping me a victim.

My point and counterpoint with God spilled over into conversations Cindy and I had. She asked me where in the Bible I was told to wait for

Dad to apologize. I attempted to correct her doctrine with the famous forgiveness conversation between Jesus and Peter. Peter had asked if the rule of thumb of forgiving seven times applied to the Lord's teaching. Jesus crushed Peter's pride when He said, "Not seven, but seventy times seven" (see Matthew 18:21-22). That conversation started with, "If my brother comes to me and asks for me to forgive him . . ."

The emphasis I gave that last line in my argument reminded me of when Cindy and I played pinochle with her parents. My father-in-law had this habit of playing his trump card on the trick with a flourish, pecking it with his forefinger and laughing. I must have looked a lot like that with my retort to Cindy's question. And I must have deflated like my father-in-law did when the next player beat him with a higher trump card. Cindy popped my bravado with, "But aren't we supposed to be living out Christ's example? He forgave us before we asked Him."

I changed the subject. I wasn't ready to move in that direction.

I cried out in my heart to the Lord that I didn't have it within me to forgive.

Jesus added emphasis to what I was going through with reminders like, "If you love Me, keep My commandments" and "Love your enemies." Paul wrote many verses about our walk as Christians and how our lives are to reflect the Lord. Yet John perhaps said it all in 1 John 2:6: "He who says he abides in Him ought himself also to walk just as He walked." My failure brought heavy conviction—not condemnation, though at times it felt like it.

As my journey continued, the Lord steered me toward two books. The title of the first one spoke directly to my known and heartfelt need: *Total Forgiveness* by R. T. Kendall. I knew this book held something for me when I read one sidebar quote: "I had to make an important decision: Which do I prefer—the peace or the bitterness?"[2]

One lesson I learned from his book became a forgiveness barometer for me. It is perhaps the greatest lesson in his book: Evaluate how you feel about bad memories and those who caused them. Do they trigger the same emotions as before? If so, forgiveness is not complete. Had I read through the book a few times, my thirty-nine-year journey might have been shortened, but it clarified and reinforced what I sensed in my heart and what I was reading in Scripture.

The second book, written by Dr. Robert S. McGee, was *The Search for Significance*. Dr. McGee revealed four lies from the enemy of our souls that we tend to live with and the truth in God's Word to defeat them. I saw them in my life as I read through the chapters. It seemed as though I had faced and had been defeated by every one of the lies:

Acceptance Through Performance—the first lie.[3] I thought I could gain acceptance, favor, and love by what I could accomplish. I purposed to make Dad, Mom, aunts, and uncles proud of my successes. Failures hit hard. I deemed my inability to compete unfair. Being unnoticed cut me the deepest. That spilled over into my Christian experience. I looked for signs of approval: answered prayers, doors opening for me, accolades from my peers. The most difficult times to walk by faith proved to be those times when I needed to sit out quietly and learn. Like the clay that is kneaded then set on the shelf, Jesus had times for me to wait. In silence. Not even His voice to sustain and encourage.

Dr. McGee explained how God does not measure performance. He fully accepted us the moment that Jesus' blood sacrificed for us is applied to our lives. The work is done, complete. I can add nothing to it.

Addiction to Approval—the second lie.[4] Seeking recognition and approval of others became such an obsession that I fit into Dr. McGee's definition of an approval addict. I needed to receive approval of others in order to feel good about myself. Lack of praise translated into rejection. I saw rejection in simple body stances or flatline comments. Criticism, no matter how constructive and encouraging, caused me to withdraw. But God's Word proclaims, "You, who once were alienated and enemies in your mind by wicked works, yet now He has reconciled in the body of His flesh through death, to present you holy, and blameless, and above reproach in His sight" (Colossians 1:21-22). I am now, through Jesus in me, fully accepted and approved. So much so that no one can pluck me from His hand: "My sheep hear My voice, and I know them, and they follow Me. And I give them eternal life, and they shall never perish; neither shall anyone snatch them out of My hand. My Father, who has given them to Me, is greater than all; and no one is able to snatch them out of My Father's hand. I and My Father are one" (John 10:27-30).

Blame Game—the third lie.[5] I knew I had good things to offer. I had my own set of valuable skills. Therefore, any rejection I perceived had to be the fault of someone else. For instance, sports never held any attraction for me because I blamed them for separating me from my guy friends when I was young. My bad feet prevented me from participating in their games during school recess. Later in life, I convinced myself that my suggestions for improvements in the workplace were rejected because higher-ups felt their authority threatened should I receive the credit for a positive change. The blame game even came between God and me as I blamed a lot of my troubles on my disability and His refusal to give me a miracle healing. Again, God's Word reminds me of the extremely high price He paid—my deserved judgment—just so He could make me His joint heir.

Accepting Shame—the fourth lie.[6] The end of compounded rejection is shame. I began to believe everyone else must be right in their assessment of me. I lacked skills in so many areas. I couldn't do many things that looked exciting. Others exceeded my best attempts at the things I felt I had mastered. Conclusion: *I am what I am and that's the end of it.* But God's Word doesn't agree with that. I have the mind of Christ (who is responsible for having created all things—with such imagination and creativity). I am a new creation (once Jesus has put His Holy Spirit in me). Nothing is impossible for God (and that includes working through me in marvelous ways, too marvelous for words). The possibilities are above all I could ask or think.

In addition to the insights these two books provided, Jesus worked on my heart attitudes apart from my relationship with Dad. Because of the lies I had believed, I had closed much of my heart to the Holy Spirit's prompting. That had to change before I could let Dad into my life.

I remember a time, about two years before Dad died and at least twenty-five years before I got my hands on those two books, when I felt none of my prayers reached beyond my bedroom ceiling. They hit it and shattered, falling on the floor around me. I spent a day fasting and praying while struggling to stay focused on things at work. Returning home that day after work, I secluded myself in our spare bedroom and knelt in more prayer, begging the Lord to speak to me. I needed to know I was not forsaken.

He startled me on many levels when He spoke to my heart. *You have an ought against someone.* (Yes, I heard the King James Version *ought*, but I knew what He meant: an offense, a grudge, anger for some perceived wrong.)

I sat up, wiping away tears of anguish. "You have been listening! Show me who it is, and I will forgive them. I'll do whatever it takes to end this silence toward me."

It's against Me.

I couldn't have been more surprised if He had slapped me. "How can that be? You see how I have cried out for Your presence. Would I do that if I were angry at You?"

You are angry that I did not heal your feet but chose for you to have surgery instead.

A fiery sword cut through me. *Guilty!*

I had been treating God in the same way I treated Dad. I had stacked up all my bad experiences in my life from having been born with club feet and considered them a serious wrong against me. David wrote in Psalm 139:13 that God formed him in the womb. So I transferred those verses to me and concluded God formed me with a disability, and then refused to heal me. That was the greater sin to me. Why shouldn't I find fault and hold a grudge against Him? Up to that moment, I didn't see that as sin.

When God called me out, I saw only the pain I had endured and not my pride judging the only Righteous Judge. But with that one argument I put forward, my blinders were removed. The sense of being a lost cause washed over me again. I wondered how long His patience toward me would last. The wave of shame gave way to His love and forgiveness that blanketed me.

That experience taught me that, from our heavenly Father's point of view, unforgiveness of any proportion has no part in His kingdom, and no sin is darker than another. This particularly applied to how I viewed my unforgiveness toward Dad and his offences to me. To God, no degrees of sin exist. He hates them all.

The two books (*Total Forgiveness* and *Search for Significance*) that God put in my hands challenged me to filter my memories through the light of what God says, not what my enemy says. As they highlighted certain truths of Scripture, I opened my heart more to letting Jesus open the wounds in my past. Deeper healing, greater trust, bottomless joy, and total forgiveness lay within sight, but still out of reach.

Through more than thirty years and at unexpected times, a memory I had either suppressed or simply forgotten jumped into my thoughts and conversation. I struggled with them. I resented having to deal with unforgiveness again. I wanted to be done with it. However, the *God-said-it, I-believe-it, that-settles-it* approach didn't work for me. I had to accept the fact I had nearly thirty years of emotional scabs to pull off to expose the wounds and receive healing.

My healing came through this slow process. God's pace gave me deeper understanding of Dad's heart, gave me my new image of him, and increased my forgiveness in ways a one-time swipe might not have done. For example, when Uncle Bob said the war changed Dad, I accepted it as fact. I wondered what event happened to make a loving father into the monster I knew. Long after Dad died, I understood it. I still didn't know the event, but the change Dad experienced received a name through my own personal experience: post-traumatic stress syndrome.

When my eldest son came home from serving in the army, I got a deeper education on what PTSD is and what it does to an individual. We could get unintentionally injured if we tried to wake Nathan with a touch or a loud noise. The fireworks around the Fourth of July holiday triggered shaking until he could convince himself he had no reason to be afraid. Later, his PTSD, the traumatic brain injury, and stress collided and rendered him unable to handle his own affairs until he could remove himself from the triggers.

Experiencing my own PTSD moment helped me realize another error I had been holding onto. Fear of what others might think of me, fear of more rejection, shame over something I had no control over— all these kept this part of the Lord's work in my life underground. In keeping my past secret, I refused to give Him glory in what He has done for me. Doing so put me into a position of resisting God and giving place to the devil. The shame I felt gave Satan a handle to grab and pull me away from more of God's grace. My purpose in sharing it now is a prayer that others will be encouraged. Tremendous freedom (and I believe better health) comes through forgiveness. And as Jesus said in Mark 10:27, "What is impossible with man is possible with God" (my paraphrase).

With each memory awakening, I asked Jesus to forgive me . . . again. He did . . . again. He is so faithful to do that. The apostle John tells us so in his first letter. God will forgive and so much more: "If we confess our sins, He is faithful and just to forgive us our sins and to cleanse us from all unrighteousness" (1 John 1:9).

Here we find the most basic principle of why the gospel is called Good News—that "while we were still sinners, Christ died for us" (Romans 5:8). We take that so lightly. We fail to consider or appreciate what it means to be a sinner before a holy, righteous God in whom there is no speck of darkness. All of us were in a state that made us His enemies— bitter, unthinkable enemies. His love is so much greater that He forgives even before we know we need His forgiveness. He reached across so great a chasm (perfection in holiness and righteousness to hearts filled with wickedness). We make excuses for going across the street, town, state, or country to ask forgiveness. More importantly, as I experienced, why do we feel we can sit in judgment and demand they ask first?

I messed up with Dad when I went to him to ask for his forgiveness. I forced his hand to ask me to forgive him. In so doing, I put my apology into question. But God's grace is so much greater than our foibles. He turned things around for me. Dad's salvation might have happened sooner but for my overstepping Jesus' instruction.

I wish I had obeyed Jesus perfectly. I've let my thoughts dance through the conversations about Jesus that Dad and I could have had. Maybe I could have learned from him how much he loved me but didn't know how to show it. How much healing could have taken place in the time he had left instead of filling my days with anxious prayers for his salvation? We could have attended worship together as I had wanted instead of worshiping at the same time separated by a grave.

In the end, God brought me to the same place. Jesus was faithful to answer my prayers. I have Dad waiting for me in heaven. I know a happy family reunion awaits where we will worship our Lord at the throne. I thank God for His mercy and patience toward me for this story to have a happy ending. I thank Him for healing my heart and memories and for the lessons He has brought me through.

Forgiveness is at the core of Christianity. Unforgiveness betrays our witness. We can't be love while holding bitterness, demanding justice, and/or seeking revenge. We are called ambassadors for the kingdom. As such we are to be an accurate representation of His nature and to function under His authority and power.

We have also been given the ministry of reconciliation. As our older Brother, Jesus has broken the trail before us to follow in His footsteps. He has foiled the snares laid before us and given us His strength when we are weak.

Everything within me says my story's ending changed when I decided to obey God and asked Dad to forgive me. A deep work began that day in my heart, and salvation and deliverance started working in Dad's.

It made little sense to me at the time. I fought it. Worse, I resented it, but I think God's greatest handywork springs out of obedience when what He asks makes no sense. Had Dad not responded to the Holy Spirit, I would still have to praise Jesus for the cleansing work He has done in my heart. Bitterness destroys a person. I've been set free from it. I'm reminded that before I asked for it, Jesus forgave me of so much. I'm thankful He took me through forgiving Dad before he knew he needed it. How awesome is the miracle of forgiveness!

CHAPTER 11

TWO NEW MEN

I am not the same man I was at the beginning of my story. While Dad didn't get the gift of more time to change, his image in my heart changed greatly, making him new. Thus, he and I are two new men. In telling his story, I sometimes still choke, and tears flow, but not from fear, anger, or pain. At times, I grieve for what Dad missed out on, what our family missed out on.

In Jesus' Sermon on the Mount, He said, "Blessed are those who mourn, for they shall be comforted" (Matthew 5:4). Looking up definitions of *blessed* and *mourn* confused me at first. *Blessed* means happy, but more than happy—superb happiness, even to the point of being giddy. *Mourn* means excessive crying, deep grief, wailing. I knew that a deep meaning lay beneath the surface of what Jesus said. As I considered the sequential order of the verses before and after, I came to understand that the grieving Jesus was encouraging us to press into referred to the impact sin has in our lives and the lives of those around us.

To the wayward child, to the homeless vet sitting on the corner, to the difficult coworker or boss, and yes, to the abuser—we must grieve instead of judge them for what sin has done and is doing in their lives. Picture them redeemed and standing beside you in worship instead of being taken away in handcuffs.

I've done that with a few people. In one instance, I had a brother in the Lord ask me in pure meekness if I had been able to pray for the offender. It was hard to confess the truth, but I eventually said no. Then he responded in a way I could not have prepared myself for. Instead of quoting verses or some well-meaning instruction, he said, "I'll pray for him on your behalf until you can."

Several days later, I was awakened from a dream where the justice I wanted was meted out by the court. I left the courtroom feeling vindicated but also empty. I got back to sleep but was awakened with a second dream in which I had my arm over the shoulder of the offender, walking with him into church and introducing him as a new brother in Christ. The joy I felt in that dream convinced me that being and proving myself right amounts to nothing compared to helping another become right with Jesus.

I've lost touch with the different ones I've had the opportunity to have a right response with, so I can't say what has happened in their lives since the events. I can only attest to the freedom from anger, bitterness, and revenge and the Lord's joy ministered into my heart and life.

With that in mind, I want to introduce you to my dad as I see him now.

Joseph A. Huff, third born of six siblings. He arrived only two days before the end of World War I. I don't know when his father stopped farming and moved into town, but the Great Depression caught them there. It hit them hard. I can still hear Dad telling Mom her family didn't have it so bad during the depression. His closing argument was always, "You were able to have milk gravy on your farm. We couldn't afford milk, so we had water gravy."

Even in the hardships, Dad was able to distract and bring a smile. Grandpa lived by the long-standing maxim that children were to be seen but not heard—especially around the dinner table. Yet Uncle Bob told me that my dad was the family clown.

Uncle Bob related how Dad always got his brothers and sisters in trouble. He would make faces or act up in some way to make the others laugh. When one could not hold it any longer and let the laughter out, Grandpa gave a fearsome reprimand to the offender with his eyes. He would then look around the table to see who had created the interruption.

Dad would be quietly eating his food with a straight face as though what had happened escaped his notice.

I could believe that of Dad because he could always keep a straight face and rarely laughed. A hilarious joke or movie scene might arouse a snicker or even an audible chuckle, but nothing more. At family reunions, the funny stories and antics came from Uncle Bob and Uncle George. I wondered how much more of a clown he had been than they were. I remember one Halloween when my uncles George and Bob got all gussied up with wigs, masks, apple-stuffed bras, and dresses to see what sort of mischief they could have with their in-laws. And, oh, how they loved to laugh. I never saw any of that in Dad. No silliness. No pranks. All about business—or drink.

Like many in rural America in the 1930s, Dad never went beyond eighth grade. Instead, he helped his dad farm after the family moved back to the old homestead. Even after Dad and Mom married, he stretched his income and his time to help his family. His dad was having health issues and could not do as much as he used to. With his youngest two still in school, Grandpa struggled earning enough to cover household expenses. Dad gave them money from time to time.

He was loyal to his parents, siblings, aunts, and uncles. He helped them when and where he could. And he was never without a job for long. When it meant income for the family, he applied his strength and skills where needed. (Grandma's champion.)

Dad farmed, worked in the oilfields during the oil boom, and later worked in the Civilian Conservation Corp (CCC) for his part in the early war effort. The CCC was part of President Roosevelt's economic boost in the depression that expanded jobs in agriculture. When the farming exemption from the draft lifted, Dad joined the army. He was almost twenty-five, married, and had a son, who was nearly two years old. His first assignment put him in the anti-aircraft division, later became a military police officer (M.P.), and ended his time in the service as a mess sergeant. For his time in the Pacific front, he received a bronze star. Dad refused to talk about his wartime experiences except for blurting out certain phrases when situations triggered a response. "I hope you never have to go through anything like what I went through."

On rare occasions, he shared snippets of his experience, such as how he disobeyed orders for the sake of starving Filipinos. "Outside the mess hall, we had slop barrels for the food scraps we threw away. No one was to be near them, but local children would dip bowls in to retrieve what they could to feed themselves or their family. When I could, I let them put their bowls under the plates I was scraping." He preferred doing that over watching them dip cups and pails into the barrels. Both actions violated his orders and would have cost him if caught.

He also told about the end of the war. His outfit boarded troop transport ships in preparation for invading Japan. They sat in the harbor a few days and then were ordered back off the ships. Orders had changed; they were to wait. Two weeks later our planes dropped the atomic bombs on Hiroshima and Nagasaki. Dad's unit then became part of the occupation force instead of the invasion force.

It's possible Dad's experiences in the war planted in him the bravery he showed when he ran toward the wrecked car many years later. He could have shrunk back as I did, but he didn't. Courage and concern for the welfare of others carried him into the menacing cloud and led him to be the essential help to a total stranger in need. It was his responsibility simply because he was there. It was the right thing to do and there was no one else to do it.

Mom always said Dad was excellent in math. Maybe that talent was at play in his car buying. He never bought the latest model car, choosing instead one that was up to two years old. I thought his selection was based on price. As I look back, I wonder if he didn't already understand what modern financial advisors and wealth builders teach. His pattern was to buy a lightly used car—one with most of its depreciation from the new price already taken off. The car he traded in would be about five years old—just about to start the season of failing systems but with many good years ahead, based on mileage. I shake my head when I think how old I was when I let that wisdom sink in. For him, it was all part of taking care of his family as best he could.

That was my dad.

Courageous, dutiful, compassionate, loyal, responsible, diligent, hard-working. I recognize all those traits in him as the Lord has given me eyes to see them.

Also loving. Dad loved me even though he didn't know how to show it, but he did most importantly in the way I needed to see it in later years. He had not learned a father's expression of love from his dad. As a result, I never knew Dad's love. But God has shown me how Dad tried showing it in his way. Opening and setting up the Monopoly game that one Christmas, the many Christmas gifts I selfishly asked for and he gave, the binoculars, the motorcycle I didn't ask for, his war keepsakes (the Japanese rifle, bayonet, and officer's sword), even allowing and encouraging my skills in pinochle. God showed me those were Dad's ways of telling me he loved me. I never understood or accepted them when I was growing up. They were lost on me—being under the weighty cloud of the victim tag—until Jesus began opening my eyes and freed me so that I am a victim no more.

I've reached a place where I have forgiven and loved him more since his death than I ever imagined. One proving evidence of that for me is that I can now sing the one verse in the song "I Have Returned" and see Dad in it.

ACKNOWLEDGMENTS

I concluded long ago that I am who I am today because of the people in my life. Whether through genetic inheritance or personal encounters, I bear some mark of difference or change. From the ancestors who were circuit-riding preachers and earlier down through the ages to my children and grandchildren, aunts and uncles, and cousins—all too many to list, thank you.

Another long list includes my Word Weavers International critique group members (my wife being one of them because she is why I started taking writing seriously) as they had to suffer through reading my early drafts. Their encouragement and insights helped more than I can express here.

Once this book was near final stage, a smaller group of friends gave their time to read the pre-published copy. As a test audience of sorts, they provided much needed comments for final adjustments and so added value.

Finally, I thank Ginger Kolbaba who in 2021 served me as my writing coach and editor, refining my efforts and making me dig deeper. She was the first person to learn many of the stories in this book. Rather than flinching, she sent me words of encouragement, believing my story needed to be told when I was ready to give up. I'm sure she would also thank my critique partners for their work, which made her work easier.

ENDNOTES

1. Chapian, Marie., Sadler, Robert. *The Emancipation of Robert Sadler: The Powerful True Story of a Twentieth-Century Plantation Slave.* United States: Baker Publishing Group, 2012.

2. R. T. Kendall, *Total Forgiveness: When Everything in You Wants to Hold a Grudge, Point a Finger, and Remember the Pain—God Wants You to Lay It All Aside* (Lake Mary, FL: Charisma, 2002), xxviii.

3. Robert S. McGee, *The Search for Significance: Seeing Your True Worth Through God's Eyes* (W Publishing, 1998, 2003), chapters 3 and 4.

4. McGee, *The Search for Significance,* chapters 5 and 6.

5. McGee, *The Search for Significance,* chapters 7 and 8.

6. McGee, *The Search for Significance, chapters 9 and 10.*

ABOUT THE AUTHOR

Charles J. Huff is a collector. In his early years, he collected antiques, but his favorite collection consists of stories: family stories, humorous stories, and faith stories. While others can list one life verse from Scripture, Charles has several, but one of his first to hold close is Psalm 119:19 "I am a stranger (sojourner) in the earth; do not hide your commandments from me." Because that has been his cry after putting his faith in Jesus Christ, Charles has tried to help others experience faith and grow in their relationship with Jesus.

Charles Huff has served as Bible teacher and minister in his church for twenty years. His devotions have appeared in www.christiandevotions.us, *The Upper Room,* and is a monthly contributor to Inspire A Fire, an on-line blogsite with potential readership above 9,000 per month. He also has articles in three anthologies: *Gifts from Heaven: True Stories of Miraculous Answers to Prayer/* "Shortest, Biggest Prayer," compiled by James Stuart Bell; *Short and Sweet Too/* "To Sleep—All Night," compiled by Susan Cheeves King; and *Short and Sweet Takes the Fifth/* "Oh, To Have Seen Him!" compiled by Susan Cheeves King.

Charles has won awards for his non-fiction articles and short stories at writers conferences.

Charles and his wife Cindy (author Cindy Ervin Huff) have five children and eight grandchildren with and additional three step-grand-children whom they love spending time with. He and his wife have traveled three times to the Philippines where they have held pastors seminars and taught in various churches, including remote mountain churches. Having a heart for helping others deepen their relationship with Jesus, Charles writes a blog he calls his Boosterclub Blog. It can be found at www.chashuff.wordpress.com. He is a charter member of Word Weavers of Aurora, Illinois, and is president of one of Word Weavers on-line critique groups.

www.ingramcontent.com/pod-product-compliance
Lightning Source LLC
Chambersburg PA
CBHW070807280326
41934CB00012B/3094